PRACTICAL LIFE STYLE

By

Ramaswamy Thanu

Printed by CreateSpace
An Amazon Company

Contents

About the Book

The book *Practical Life Style* opens the door to health and happiness and welcomes all human beings desirous of living a healthy, happy and productive life. It contains the essence of wisdom of the past with techniques adapted and molded to the needs of the present. The gateways to disease depict the major unhealthy ways of living to which the present generation has fallen. It
explains the means of attaining happiness enjoying better physical and mental health. A solution is suggested for resolving marital conflicts, facing misfortunes and overcoming depression. Great emphasis is laid on the lessons that can be learnt usefully from Nature for ones happiness. A calm and positive approach is outlined for facing death which is an inevitable event in man's life. It concludes with a note on the importance of loving all for one's own happiness and for the welfare, happiness and prosperity of the world. Believing in the maxim 'small is beautiful' the author has condensed so much wisdom and suggestions in so few pagers to benefit so many readers. The contents reflect largely the authors own experience and conviction which makes him feel young even in old age.

PRACTICAL LIFE STYLE

1. Gateway to Disease

Man is a unique creation in this planet. But in this vast universe where even the Milky Way is one among the 100 billion galaxies, and the sun, one in 100 billion stars in its parent galaxy, where and what is he in size, strength and power. . Though he has great achievements and material prosperity, is he really happy despite his unique discriminating faculty? Can he be really happy? Yes, if he acquires transformation technology of self-management.

Why do we need this? Wasteful knowledge depletes energy through pursuing a constellation of desires. Confusion brings tension and stress making one eligible for chronic diseases. Such men live in dissatisfaction and happiness eludes them. Like the caterpillar that takes the thread from its own mouth, builds its cocoon and at last finds itself caught inside, many bind themselves by own actions. Such rudderless performance results from imbalance in the body, mind and intellect system. Expectations grow fast and many remain unfulfilled. The enormous intangible resource of talent and energy within man is untapped and potential not realized for benefit and happiness.

: There are individuals who don't know what they want in life. They engage in some activity, which gives them money, and they go on slogging for years. Their ambition is confined to eating, sleeping, merry making, visiting places, rearing children, educating them and finally retiring from job and from the world. If you ask them what they have left behind as contribution, the answer can be found only in the toilets. They have left tons of current deposits. Of course this is an exaggeration. But to understand what happens with most individuals and what approach is helpful, this example is enough.

Let us consider an illustration. This is applicable to all human beings, man or woman. A man gets up at 6 am. He does his morning duties in hurry and reaches office by 9 am. He does work the meaning of which he does not know. His lunch is at 1 p.m and after work he returns in the evening by 6 p.m. He goes to bed at 11 p.m. He always complains of lack of time for any important work. Does he ask what he has done with the time available? Does he ask what he has done with the funds available? Let us ask a few questions to ascertain his contribution to society and to his family.

Everyone wants to maintain a trim figure and struggle for weight loss if they measure high in the weighing scale. But they let loose the reins on their gluttony when they see delicious food. They overload the belly, consume the wrong type of foodstuff akin to filth and do least exercise except probably that intended for breeding. They yearn for an athletic figure but end up with a gorilla shape.

It is sad that many men and women ignore wake up calls. Eating junk food becomes a regular habit and hobby. These creatures start growing sideways. For every inch of such growth they add five pounds to their already bulging body. They find themselves immobile and move like a baby elephant. Clothes and innerwear take odd shapes adequate enough to accommodate a hippo. These humans get frustrated but do nothing to improve the situation. When they reach their forties they suddenly realize that overweight poses threat to longevity. They are unable to live an active life or engage in physical activity. They try short cuts by way of medicines but what gets reduced is their bank balance and not body weight

Some people are obese by heredity. They eat mercilessly as if they were filling a garbage bag.

They are highly automated individuals getting everything on their seats. Eating or drinking is done to taste and impulse and not out of considerations of health and wellbeing.

Sticking to a routine for well-being is difficult for most people. Very few people are committed for the long-term to healthy eating, exercise, and good habits. Our lifestyles and bad habits often stand in the way. For those severely out of shape, beginning and sticking to new lifestyle changes can be much more difficult than for a person who has a few kgs. to lose. However, it's more crucial to commit to change if a person really wants to prolong his life span and enjoy life more

Stress is a major contributing factor to coronary artery disease, cancer, respiratory disorders, accidental injuries, cirrhosis of the liver and suicide. It is the response of the human body to any physical, emotional or intellectual demands. We can't eliminate stress. But we can do a better job in managing it. Managing stress requires following a healthy diet, regular exercise, and budgeting time for uninterrupted relaxation. Symptoms of stress are different for different persons. Some common signs are: too much excitement, impatience, disturbed sleep and exhaustion.

Almost every human being has felt the burden of worries some time or other. In some cases people constantly worry and others less frequently. They worry about persons, events, and things; Worry is a painful mental condition full of mental uneasiness and agitations. It saps all energy and leads to mental and physical illness of various kinds. It blocks clear thinking.

Commonly observed physical symptoms of stress include muscular rigidity, headaches, low back pain, insomnia and high blood pressure. These symptoms may manifest themselves psychologically as irritability, anxiety, poor concentration, mental confusion, poor judgment, frustration and anger. Some people with chronic illness may find that the symptoms of their illness flare up under excessive stress. The complexity of stress management is that, when dealing with stress generating events that are enjoyable one may not always realize how stressed one feels until one experience serious stress symptoms.

A person purchases goods which are not of immediate use and which satisfy his vanity. Soon he is overpowered by the presence of better and more expensive items in his friend's home. This tempts him to procure those items. He tries to keep up with the Joneses. There is more income, more goods and services but no peace of mind.

What has he done? He has purchased goods and services. But he has purchased misery also along with them. Had he not purchased such goods and services he would not have been compelled to look for storage space or devote time for maintenance. Such resources and time could be utilized for more productive purposes.

. He looks dull though he is very busy. He tries hard to accumulate more and more material things. He has no place to store them. He does not have time to keep them in good condition. The articles suffer neglect and damage. He finds replacement. This cycle goes on. But all along he has no peace of mind. His mind is always agitated. This is more so for a person operating on a tight budget.

Everybody wants steady material progress and comforts. Each one of us wants happiness. We work hard to produce articles, gadgets and services for maximum comfort, convenience and enjoyment. Parameters are framed based on the quantum of these factors coming in our possession and we call this progress. We say we have achieved a lot. This we call our mastery over nature. We eat, build, live, enjoy, breed and sleep. This cycle goes on and every day we wake up with the hope of widening the circle of happiness including many more things and articles in its fold. Then where do we go.

Greed is nothing but the tendency to possess more and more of goods and services whether we need them or not. The purpose is only to impress others and to show our vanity. Do we expect to carry along with us the things we accumulate when the last tick of the clock ticks us away forever?

Progress leaps forward. Every one counts wealth, riches and money. There is surplus money everywhere and men go after chasing investment channels for multiplying wealth. They accumulate. But then comes a disastrous moment. Suddenly the market crashes. The downfall starts. And leaders all over the world call for austerity and adjustments. They call for sacrifices. They fear and face massive unemployment and steep fall in income and standards of living. The heavy blow of the recession consequent to the unchecked progress makes us the laughing stock of wise men. We discover that we have been unwise. That is the wisdom of being foolish. We allowed the senses to rule over us and not the brain. We allowed greed to overtake us and our sanity. The downfall seems a break less journey. So many brakes are applied but they all jam. We sit in solitude and lament over the tragedy.

For discharging one's duty in life to various persons if these things are required we can understand it. But this is not the case always. How can we continue to amass goods and add to our comforts when billions of our brethren are steeped in poverty and misery? Take the case of people in some countries of Africa and Asia. Should we not make a beginning to think how best we can contribute? Ask questions like the following.

Have I:

Utilized time productively?

Done the job encrusted to him in the best possible manner?

Conserved his energy?

Time for spending with his family?

Done any good work to help others?

Lived happily?

Do I:

Take the family out daily for relaxation?

Share the household work?

Read self-improvement books?

Have peace of mind?

Am I

At peace with myself?

Happy

Have we respected the wisdom of the ages? The old men of vision had great concern for the whole of humanity. They lived simple lives and emphasized on service to others. Their example was of one of sacrifice and service. Now our champions of individualism and material progress substituted it by self aggrandizement, self enrichment and self above service. Many social organizations silently implanted this philosophy with the result wealth of all types including filth was produced and amassed. This was far beyond the basic requirements of individuals. Then the bang was felt.

Often we come across people who always complain of something or other. They say they have no time even for any essential activity. They complain about inability to make both ends meet, time squeeze, mounting debt, inadequate income, obesity, inability to keep up with the Joneses etc. The list is only illustrative. Always their conversation brings in some complaint or other and centre on what they lack in comparison to their colleagues or neighbors. We can understand if this is a temporary feature or a genuine complaint. Often it is not.

Such individuals make themselves miserable. They can never be at peace with themselves. This state of declaring a war with oneself makes others also miserable. Thus they radiate unhappiness all around. They waste considerable energy. If only they use such energy for solving their problems it would have been understandable and worthwhile. They do not make any attempt to solve the problem. The problem remains. The result is they always brood over unattainable things.

If they get someone to talk they unleash all their grievances on them as if the listener can help to find a solution. They forget that they themselves are responsible for such a misery. Lack of time is due to absence of priority for doing various activities. Unnecessary and unproductive activity makes serious inroads into their time. They spend more hours in sleep and waste the waking hours on futile pursuits.

They do not have a budget and control over expenditure and hence they are unable to make both ends meet. Here we talk about persons who are well of and belong to the middle class in respect of income and status. They do not analyze their daily activities and are poor in time management. Their greed goes on unabated that they accumulate goods and gadgets indiscriminately which drain their valet and create congestion in their homes and belly. Thus they waste lot of mental energy by complaining about things and facilities they lack.

The disease with modern civilization is indiscriminate lopsided material progress. Happiness is associated with increasing possessions and comforts. There is no end to this. Thus we invite restlessness of the mind, which is the root cause of our entire mental imbalance that is unhappiness. We know that worldly possessions do give feeling of satisfaction and comfort. But we must realize that such satisfaction is purely temporary and it disappears when the object or comfort is absent or when craving for another object or comfort arises.

Detailed studies of hundreds of patients and research findings reveal that even a small lateral expansion of the belly with extra fat and a sedentary lifestyle can increase risk of heart disease. Abnormal overweight can raise the threat of heart disease. It is not necessary to be obese to have heart ailments.

.

Sticking to a routine for well-being is difficult for most people. Very few people are committed for the long-term to healthy eating, exercise, and good habits. Our lifestyles and bad habits often stand in the way. For those severely out of shape, beginning and sticking to new lifestyle changes can be much more difficult than for a person who has a few kgs. to lose. However, it's more crucial to commit to change if a person really wants to prolong his life span and enjoy life more.

There are inbuilt obstacles to achieve success. A thyroid malfunctioning hinders metabolism, and affects treatment for weight reduction. Individual circumstances influence schedule flexibility. But these should not be used as excuses.

Men want to satisfy their wants. Wants and desires multiply They are the indiscriminate offspring of the mind .When they are satisfied at the lowest level more and more desires and wants manifest and demand fulfillment. This becomes greed. The nature of greed and its growth are like pouring ghee into fire. The intensity becomes great. When resources are not available to satisfy greed, crooked methods are sought. Greed commands resources and this need not be based on priority. So resources are cornered by people who perpetuate and promote greed. Though we may call many of them entrepreneurs, many turn out to be thieves of society.

When the tendency to satisfy greed becomes predominant in society such a society adopts all means fair and foul to muster resources. This leads to extensive borrowing since own resources may be inadequate. Excessive borrowing creates a situation that repayment of loans becomes difficult and default occurs. This sets in motion a chain reaction and the economy collapses causing fall in employment and rise in economic misery. The lone culprit is greed.

"We live under severe stress. We are susceptible to heart diseases at a very young age. Most of the time people start smoking to get over stress," According to a survey, over 3.5 million Indians, 50 percent of them from productive age groups, will die of heart diseases by 2010"Intake of food rich in fats and carbohydrates, smoking, stress and lack of exercise are some of the factors leading to cardiovascular diseases," This state is threatened when unsatisfied desires constantly haunt us. We are haunted by cravings for things and this wrecks our peace of mind.

2. Happiness in Daily Life

Happiness is the goal of all human beings. It is a state of mind. It is an intangible gift the value and benefits of which cannot be determined, described and discussed. It is a realized experience. One may have considerable wealth, comforts and other resources and yet feel miserable. On the other hand we find people with meager resources but are happy. They are always cheerful. They have enthusiasm. Everyone who comes into contact with such people feels happy. The association is remembered and sought after. This is a blessing, which cuts across all economic borders.

 One may have a lot of wealth and resources and yet be miserable. The whole lifetime of man is devoted in pursuit of acquiring material goods and other possessions. Temporarily they feel happy. But desires for other goods and services arise and the pursuit again starts. We also find people with meager resources who are happy. The never complain. They are never agitated. They radiate a feeling of contentment, which is their valuable possession. All human beings want a comfortable and happy life, which is a mental condition free from stress and tensions.

.. A man becomes happy when he is contented or at peace with himself Happiness is an enjoyable feeling, a state of mind .It may originate from wealth, possession, or, a state of enjoyment and contentment. This means a variety of things to many. People think acquisition of material objects of consumption; comforts, convenience, riches, wealth, status, power, pleasure, fame, recognition, marriage, job etc. will give real happiness. They run after these ephemeral attractions not knowing their transient nature. In fact this hot pursuit of happiness becomes elusive and disappointing. Every individual seeks these attractions. Yet, true love and happiness are privileges enjoyed only by a few.

For most people happiness lies in achievements, satisfaction of ego, success and getting an edge over competitors, obtaining material goods, and similar factors. We satisfy our egos, believe in its demands and wishes, and revel in its achievements. Elimination of ego, generous acts of love, contemplation of love of God in our hearts, wiping of hatred from our minds, forgiveness, sacrifice, and pursuit of spirituality, among others leads us to the path of perennial love and happiness.

Love and Happiness are interrelated and inseparable. Genuine acts of love lead to lasting happiness. This means showering unselfish love on our loved ones and helping them always with true love in our hearts. Happiness depends upon love-the divine feeling that takes us closer to God and all our fellow beings. With love in our hearts, we can be at peace and at harmony with others and ourselves. The pursuit of unselfish love, generosity, spirituality, gratification, and serenity results in a change in our attitude too. This change in attitude makes us realize real happiness. The intense feeling of love for God, for our close ones, and fellow-beings helps in lighting the lamp of divine happiness in this world. Love and happiness form an integral part of our life and exist as the core of our existence.

The secret of happiness is to broaden our horizons and to welcome people and their beliefs into our world with love and understanding .A happy person is not one in a certain circumstances, but rather one with certain attitudes. The foolish man seeks happiness far away whereas the wise finds it under his feet. Money, resources, and hopes are not essential to be happy. Yet one can be the happiest person alive. He is the happiest man irrespective of being king or peasant, who finds peace at home.

Happiness is an enjoyable feeling that everyone wants and cherishes cutting across all borders. One may be immensely rich, yet feel miserable. In reality pursuit of happiness from material objects and comforts, name and fame at some stage becomes elusive and disappointing. If possessions make us happy their absence makes us unhappy. The same event gives happiness to one and unhappiness to another. . The state of mind without excitement and depression ensures constant peace. We can attain this. It is a question of cultivating the right attitude towards life, events and persons. Attitude plays an important role in ensuring happiness.

Here learning to live in the present becomes important. The past is gone and future is yet to unfold. We have no control over these two periods. Worry causes mental agitations and unhappiness. We can overcome this state if we are not preoccupied with the actions of the past and anxieties about the future.

The human mind, a ten billion dollar gift, is a powerful and wonderful asset. Air cannot be tied with a rope, so is the mind. It can lift you to great heights depending on how you use and control it. The mind needs to be steady. Entertaining noble and exalted thoughts helps to achieve this. Thoughts of friendship, mercy and joy pacify the mind. Such a mind does not vacillate. This is strengthened by meditation. Think of the vast universe, the ocean and the mountain we see. Here mentally chanting the name of the Lord is greatly helps. This does not allow entry of disturbing thoughts. We can work with greater efficiency.

No doubt possessions and wealth are necessary for a comfortable life. But they should be for our needs and not greed. Decisions based on needs alone give you lasting happiness and a sustainable life style. Greed fuels corrupt practices. Nothing makes us more fortunate than the opportunity of serving others. We forget our problems when immersed in the work of helping fellow beings. Remember that the human body is an amazing creation of love and affection. No joy is greater than that of loving others Evidence suggests love needs to be brought into the health care system.

A healthy body is essential for happiness. Food, exercise and recreation in moderate doses yield good results. Such a person enjoys tranquility of mind. Like the naked flame of a candle, well protected in a place where air cannot disturb, and doesn't flutter, in a mind full of optimism anxiety to search for temporary pleasures does not arise. Such a person is unmoved by the greatest tragedy.

Spiritual progress reduces insecurity. Integration of breathing with awareness of the self is what yoga teaches. It combines abdominal and thoracic breathing. This increases the intake of oxygen and helps in controlling breath. Think of prayer as self discipline. A simple prayer "May there be peace and happiness to all creations in the Universe" will bring happiness. This fuses our mind with the Almighty for some time. After prayer we get tears of happiness. Positive thinking is a blessing and praying for the welfare of all humanity improves our mental health. Nature, the animals and trees, teach a lot if we carefully observe, listen and care for them. Certainly we owe them a duty, by way of gratitude, something in return so that posterity will remember us in great esteem. Thus practiced, self-management becomes a reality.

Life style is an important ingredient of happiness. As we grow and advance in age we can reflect on our experience, observe others and learn. This reinforces a strong feeling in us that there are people who are, healthy and free from worries.

Let us take an example of one who benefited from such a life style. Henry. 80, is engaged as a freelance writer. Even in his early twenties he was wedded to a concept of happiness as that which gives peace of mind. Anything, in conflict with this criterion he discarded. He gave up lucrative jobs and assignments because they had an unsettling effect on his happiness. .He chose to be self-employed and lived a life of his own for forty years.

There is an old adage 'early to rise and early to bed makes a man healthy, wealthy and wise'. Fully believing in this maxim, he wakes up at 4 am regularly, sits on the bed for a few minutes praying. After a wash he meditates for twenty minutes. He consumes a full glass of water. This is followed by a cup of tea after which he goes for a long walk covering 4 miles leaving my home at 5.15 am. He returns by 6.45 am.

He meets a few friends who also regularly walk on his way. Without reducing the speed they discuss some current topic and a few anecdotes generating spontaneous laughter. On return he attends to routine household work and performs yogic exercises 30 minutes.

He listens to good classical music whenever he gets time. After bath he prays for 40 minutes .The mind becomes calm and serene. Later he has his vegetarian breakfast. Writing and reading are confined to self-improvement books, scriptures that deal with values and the quintessence of ancient wisdom.

By 1PM he takes pure vegetarian lunch. From 2 PM he has a nap for forty-five minutes then does some light reading till 5 p.m. Shopping is done on some days for an hour in the forenoon or evening avoiding peak traffic. By 6 in the evening he takes bath. He watches TV for news and for some interesting educative program, by 7.30 PM he takes dinner and by 9.30 PM goes to sleep. This daily routine is normally adhered to even when he goes abroad.

His weight remains constant for thirty-five years at 145 lbs. for a height of 5'10". Yogic exercises with proper breathing take 30 minutes. Deep inhaling increases large intake of oxygen. Powerful exhaling expels the impurities inside the body. This is done several times in the morning during the exercise session. It keeps the body trim and agile. He got rid of backache completely through yogic exercise and is thus free from joint pains, which normally invade persons of his age. The stamina gives him capacity to take-up hard work.

The life style and daily routine stood him in good stead when he undertook the Mountain tour covering 1700 miles by road along the narrow paths of the mountains. He could withstand the rigors of the climate as well as the jerks and jolt of the journey- all thanks to the daily routine.

His core philosophy is to be happy. This is ensured by my faith in three principles. The first is contentment. Secondly he adopts the attitude of never complaining. Thirdly belief and practice in the philosophy of 'never live to impress others'. He keeps worry at a distance.

His actions are deeply rooted in core values and spiritual strength. He attends spiritual discourse and reads spiritual books. His children and grandchildren when living with him join in prayers daily.

Enlightened people at times are wise enough to take a resolution to reduce weight and live a healthy life. They develop an optimistic outlook towards life, environment and events. They try to maintain cheerfulness, introduce diet and exercise.

A senior citizen came on an eight-week holiday to America. Far away from home in India, he had doubts whether it would be possible for him to maintain his calm and happy state of mind, which he has been cherishing for many years. However, soon after arrival he discovered, for it is possible to live without any basic change in the daily routine. He could design his time and day to fit in with his basic objective of being happy. It proved to be an enlivening and enriching experience preserving the peace which he treasured most.

Overcoming the jet lag, daily he gets up at 5 a.m brushes his teeth and gulp a glass of cold water. Prayer, followed by reading of scriptures for forty-five minutes, is the next event. He performs his regular physical exercise consisting of various postures of yoga for the next forty minutes. This is done with rhythmic breathing, which tones up the system. Resting for fifteen minutes he goes for a long walk at 7 a.m with his wife, inside the subdivision of Cobb County along the side path enjoying and appreciating the sight of beautiful tall trees skirting the roads, backyard of homes, the colorful gardens and well-laid lawns on either side. To match the distance of four miles which he daily covered in his home land, he goes round the cull de sacs in the entire subdivision, walk up to the exit road leading to the highway, return and complete one full round of the subdivision. The weather and breeze add to his pleasant feeling and well - being.

Residents passing by wave their hands and children wait for the school bus. This sight gives a feeling of friendliness and broadens his smile. The terrain with ups and downs is beautifully landscaped. The environment is pollution free bestowing the gift of fresh air. Though he is told about the threat of pollen allergy, he is spared, probably because of the immunity developed. The walk last an hour and by 8 am he returns home.

After tea he scans through the Newspaper, note some topics for further detailed reading, for twenty minutes. Finishing bath he has breakfast by 9.30 am. This consists of cereals or bread and fruits.

He has been maintaining his weight around 145 lbs for his height of 70 inches, for the last 30 years. The variation rarely is 2 lbs and is brought back to normal by physical exercise. He takes care of his diet. After breakfast for two hours he reads newspaper, a few pages of books on great leaders and astronomy. At 1 p.m he eats pure vegetarian lunch followed by 45 minutes' nap. In the afternoon he works on the computer, developing articles centered on creativity and reflections on experience. While at home he spends time with grandchildren for an hour

In the evening he watches TV for news and educative entertainment. Some reading follows dinner at 8 p.m, and he goes to sleep by 10.pm. He enjoys undisturbed sleep. On days at home this is his routine. Even when he goes out for visiting tourist spots in and around Georgia the practice of prayer, physical exercise, and diet are rigorously maintained, advancing the time when required.

During weekends he goes out to important places of tourist interest. A few of them are the Lost Sea Mountain, Rocky City, Callaway Gardens, Stone Mountain Park, Nashville Temple, Atlanta temple, Ruby Falls and Amicalola Waterfalls. Here the mind merges with the wonders of nature, the handiwork of nature carving out millions of intricate beautiful designs in rocks. The mind is fully engaged in full appreciation of the marvelous Mother Nature and the glory of God. Adherence to physical exercise, mental discipline, and positive attitude helps considerably.

A decade ago he had the fortune to go on a pilgrimage to some of the holy shrines in the Himalayas and walk 14 kms each way in a mountainous terrain at a height of 14000 feet along a four feet rough track without any discomfort and illness. This experience gave him the strength and stamina to move around places. His stay in

USA helps to maintain the chain of happiness unbroken and by the grace of God this will hopefully continue for some years. Every moment he remembers God for the mercy showered, reinforcing faith in Him and the values enriching human life.

We all agree on one point that all human beings want to be happy? It gives us a pleasant feeling from which we would not like to return. The mind is free from agitations and full of joy. There are no cravings.

We will find the state of contentment keeps us in balance. This arises from developing a detached view of objects, events and actions. Such an attitude convinces us that there is no sorrow in this world. Sorrow is only a creation of the mind. Instead of understanding happiness as something, which gives a ripple of pleasure in the body or satisfaction in the mind, realize it as calmness arising from a mind rooted in a steady peaceful feeling. The same object gives one happiness and sorrow to others. It is the value one assigns to it. We realize that worldly objects do not have any quality to cause happiness or sorrow. It is our attitude and attachment to them that makes the difference. If we accept this concept of happiness then life becomes very enjoyable.

We thus find it useful to establish ourselves firmly in this concept of happiness. This requires mind control for which meditation is helpful. The mind is a monkey and if let loose lit will work havoc. The method of taming the mind is to develop the right attitude towards the world of objects. This will be conducive to maintain our peace of mind. Meditation, over period of time ensures elimination of all unwanted thoughts and focuses the mind on something lofty and noble.

Contentment brings peace to us internally. This gets reflected in our relationship with others. We can live according to the principle of sustainability of the environment. We will never complain for the lack of anything. We feel happy over what we have and will not crave for unattainable things. We give up the unhealthy habit of comparing our plight with others in matters of position and wealth. Thus we avoid being restless .We live for ourselves and not to impress others.

We will be considerate to others by loving them. The contented mind releases considerable energy to do our work. We do work as our duty with dedication and love others for love's sake. Our faith in God helps us to do any work as an offering to Him. We remain calm and happy. This wave of happiness and love engulfs our family and ultimately the society. We collectively can create a happy society free from strife and conflict. This is what we have to achieve.

A contented mind free of turbulence helps positive thinking. We desire only those objects and comforts, which constitute our basic needs. If acquisition of a thing causes unhappiness or disturbance we will avoid it. We realize, more than money, power or wealth, it is peace of mind that is important. We get firmly established in this thought and would not like to get away from it for it gives us peace. If this is prolonged it becomes bliss which is the extreme form of happiness.

This facilitates clear thinking. Our decisions will be sound, positive and productive. Energy is utilized productively and for our own benefit as well as for others. For this we will keep the body fit. We will maintain the sense organs in the best possible manner. Conservation of energy will lead us to realize more of the secrets of good health particularly through yogic exercises with breathing.

Happiness is to be experienced within. Contentment ensures mental state free from complaints,' non-comparison' with others and living in the present without brooding over things. If we develop this approach we will always be happy. No storm can rattle us. Our acts, events and consequences will be better appreciated. We will find life enjoyable and always be happy. There will be no misery or sorrow. We stop making ourselves miserable or invite sorrow because of our right approach to life and its problems. Contentment certainly is the key to happiness.

Thus the bane of society is greed and if we want to improve society and its economic condition we must curb greed. Greed results in wastage of resources. The recent stock market crash and global meltdown confirm this phenomenon.

The global melt down of the last decade had its origin in human greed which prompted individuals to acquire assets even at the risk of heavy borrowing. Banks welcomed borrowers to further their business. This led to business boom and later a bubble burst. We are yet to recover from the onslaught of this big hit. Share markets crashed. Banks collapsed .This resulted in loss of millions of jobs. Loss of income caused proliferation of misery. Economic theory based on multiplicity of desires and wants can only offer a faulty structure with loose foundation.

How long it will last is any body's guess. How far can the wants theory of progress go?

Are not resources cornered and wasted?

Are there not priorities for human existence? Why not upgrade human values which will definitely scale down greed and ensure better standards of living for all instead of extreme happiness for a few and acute misery for many. Controlling greed is the function of controlling the mind with the power of the intellect. If our educational system can achieve this in a decade steadily we will definitely march towards stable progress without tears. Let us start building up a global value system relinquishing greed. Let us not salute greed as an engine of economic progress

Worst of situations do not deter some persons from remaining in a totally detached and relaxed state of mind. They serve as role models for others because they radiate joy and enthusiasm. It is easy for them to win over others and earn their love and affection. They are unconcerned about the adverse reactions and they remain cool. This is a rare quality. Only a few persons are blessed with this trait. We have a few illustrations to understand such persons and benefit. from them.

Person A appears for an interview for a post in the army. He could not join for the simple reason he did not qualify. After some time one of his friends asked him.

Mr. A. What happened to your interview?

A replied: I was selected but asked not to come.

***

In another case a friend borrowed A's cycle and had a jolly ride. On the way the cycle met with a mishap and fell down. The handle bar was damaged and brakes got twisted. The matter was reported to the owner. Then A said: Don't worry. It will only improve the condition of the cycle .You have achieved which I could not for quite some time. Thank you.

***

A asks B for lending his cycle for an hour. Though A is a close friend, B is reluctant to give since the cycle belongs to another friend. He explains the position, excuses himself giving valid reasons.

A is adamant. He says" I am asking you for the cycle exactly for the same reason. If it were yours I would not have asked. Since it is someone else's I am asking because any damage caused would be his worry.

***

Person B has a medical checkup. The doctor observes three blocks in his arteries. He advises to have a bypass surgery. The cost of the surgery is $25000.When the doctor conveys this patent reacts:

"I am not worth $25000. Hence I don't propose to have this surgery"
. He lives even after 15 years.

***

A friend asks B about his post and perquisites. He adds that he has been extremely lucky to get the job and wonders how B got it despite having interviewed by the tough minded Director.

B replies: The Director knows he can get a more qualified person on a lower salary for my post. But he also knows the same is applicable to his post as well.

3. Physical Health

The human body is the greatest gift of God. This body is a holy temple in which the Lord resides. You have a mind, intellect and the senses. You must keep these instruments of knowledge and action in perfect condition. For this you have to practice mind control through meditation.

Walking

Francis Bacon, while talking about death said long ago "Men fear death just like children fear to walk in darkness". In the present context we can say" men fear to walk when they own a car". Taking it further we find men forget their legs when they land in a car. This exempts those who regularly take to walking for health and happiness. Walking is a low-impact exercise. It is the easiest exercise one could undertake. Some start with 2 kms a day and increased gradually to 6 kms. In a month they lose 2-5 kgs. This gives confidence and encouragement.

This exercise is accessible to all. It is safe, simple and suitable for all people who want to be more active. It brings several benefits. It lowers (LDL) cholesterol (the "bad" cholesterol); raises (HDL) cholesterol (the "good" cholesterol) lowers blood pressure, reduces risk of diabetes, reduces or manages your weight and helps to stay strong and physically fit. It helps to trim one's waistline, improve health and to regain health after illness. It is good for one's feeling of wellbeing.

People are aware about causes of increasing incidence of cardiovascular diseases. It is high time we started taking care of ourselves.": "Make walking part of life. It need not be a morning walk."Design a diet chart and adhere to it. Have fixed time for meals and diet should contain a combination of vitamins, proteins and essential minerals. Take packed lunch from home for office and avoid eating outside; walk after every meal; go by the stairs, avoid the lift. If you follow these simple rules of healthy life you will be richly rewarded with a life of longevity and happiness. There is no doubt about this,

Medical Journals publish tips for exercise and fitness, Body Mass Index calculator to keep track of how one is faring. In addition to the action mentioned earlier, some websites provide exercise tips that can help keep heart problems at bay. Of course, all the general medical websites propagate the benefits of exercise. Heart healthy exercise may be a key in warding off osteoarthritis, a "major cause of disability among adults over the age of 50."

Reports say that those who walk regularly have less incidence of cancer, heart disease, stroke, diabetes and other killer diseases. They live longer, get mental health and spiritual benefits.

While there are several benefits as stated above somehow

people do not take to walking seriously except when they are hit by a serious illness or health problem Such people walk under doctor's advice and not out of considerations or passion for keeping physically fit.

The best time to walk is in the early hours of the morning when there is little traffic and when air is fresh. The weather will be pleasant and invigorating. Many may not have time to walk in the morning. For them evening is the alternative. But the traffic and pollution will be adverse factors.

Walking is beneficial if one maintains the correct posture and does breathing in a manner to increase oxygen intake. It is advisable to walk with the belly drawn out while inhaling and drawn in while exhaling. This will help to take more of oxygen and leave out all impurities. The route chosen is very important to get the best results for walking. A level road is ideal. The surface should be uniform and even. Parks with walking tracks are good. One can take several rounds. Keeping the health condition in mind one can chose the route and the duration. People walk alone or in company of friends. Company removes boredom and provides relaxation. But conversation should not reduce the speed and make it more for chatting than for health benefits. Exchange of experience and funny episodes are great advantages while walking in a group. These provide laughter and acts as a health medicine.

There are many occasions when people while walking, when their minds are fresh, discuss about ideas, events, and actions of individuals. If the group consists of enlightened individuals the ambiance triggers creativity and give rise to wonderful ideas. Many articles and books have been the outcome of such interchange of ideas. These ideas are developed and have found expression in the form of books. There are several live examples in support of this.

However, an element of caution is necessary while walking. Those who walk before day break will find it useful to wear white dress so that persons coming from the opposite direction can easily identify and avoid collision. Dark colored dress reduces visibility and creates problems of identifying individuals. Light colored dress will be conducive to better visibility when the light is dim. A good pair of sports shoes will be very useful to facilitate speedy and easy movement without blisters. In chilly weather it is advisable to wear a cap to protect the head. The ears could be plugged with a soft cloth or cotton. These precautions will help to escape from cold.

There is danger of being hit by a speeding vehicle. In the early mornings traffic is less and drivers have a tendency to speed. Those not familiar with the road layout may sometimes run into posts, trees and pedestrians causing loss of life or injury. So one who walks has to be careful .It is safe to keep to the extremes of the road. It is also necessary to respect elders who take to walking for keeping physically fit. They may have problems of losing balance and slipping or fall. They may need help and young walkers have to be considerate to such persons. Conversation should be interesting rather than gossip or cynicism or playing a blame game. Morning is conducive to creativity and the occasion should be used to do creative thinking and relaxation. Care of the fellow traveler is a must .If these safeguards are observed walking becomes purposeful, enjoyable and beneficial to many.

Everyone needs good health. The constituents of good health consist of mental and physical health.

Breath

Breath is the essence of existence and life. Over 99% of our energy and oxygen come from breathing. Most diseases are caused or aggravated by poor breathing. When we breathe we inhale and exhale. While inhaling we let in oxygen, which is essential for sustaining life. When we exhale we leave out carbon did oxide, which our lungs send out along with all impurities. Proper breathing increases our lung capacity. In human beings the maximum lung capacity is attained in the late twenties. Thereafter it declines. So it becomes important to take appropriate action to improve breathing capacity and to realize the maximum potential.

Though breathing is very important, often we forget how to breathe properly and to derive maximum benefits. Normally when a person inhales he contracts the belly and when he exhales the belly expands. This is the wrong way of breathing. The right method is the reverse of this. This means inhaling is accompanied by expansion of the belly and exhaling by contraction. The correct method is to inhale with expanding belly and exhale with contracting it. The expanding belly increases intake of oxygen. When this process takes place lot of air is taken in through inhaling. A deep breath allows more oxygen to be pumped in and sent to all cells in the body. During exhaling all impurities within are flushed out. In such a practice of breathing the stomach muscles expand and contract and it helps to crush all excess fat.

In general the right method of breathing is not learnt at an early stage. Therefore the full potential of the lung capacity is not realized. Most of us practice wrong method of breathing even during the later years. We don't devote adequate attention to learn the right method in inhaling and exhaling. We hardly realize 20 to 30% of our potential when we thus breathe. We tend to be easy victim to diseases and our resistance becomes weak to ward of diseases. Hypertension is one of the diseases caused by incorrect breathing.

The correct method of breathing ensures a healthy life. To enhance the benefits we can inhale and exhale according to the principles involved in *pranayama*. This is nothing but control of breath. We close the right nostril with the thumb of the right hand and inhale through the left. Then we hold breath for a specific period by blocking both nostrils with the fingers and exhale through the right nostril (which is closed.). One method of doing this given below; while inhaling through the left nostril draw in air to full capacity of lungs for four seconds. Then we retain this for sixteen seconds blocking both nostrils and exhale slowly in eight seconds by releasing the right nostril. Reversing the process through each nostril in turn makes one cycle. The nostril through which we inhaled becomes the one through which we exhale in the reverse process. Practicing this daily brings lot of good. We can do this slowly and gently. Initially five rounds can be done and this can be gradually increased to ten or twenty or more depending on the comfort with which one is able to do. The technique of breathing and *pranayama* helps to integrate the mind, brain and body.

Breathing is part of Yoga postures. Yoga means integration of breathing with the awareness of the self, the soul of man. This increases the intake of oxygen and help in controlling breath. In asana of relaxation and inverted poses, we engage in abdominal breathing. Yoga, pranayama, vegetarian food with low fat and salt, regular physical exercise, eschewing totally alcohol and tobacco, together with compassion for all living beings help considerably in avoiding or reducing the impact of coronary artery disease. Life style modifications with a stress on tranquility of mind are the best insurance against major illness. Regular practice goes correct breathing will definitely bring you better health calmness of mind harmony and life balance. It is worth the effort. This is certain and proved by experience.

It is a remarkable feature of life that time tested simple but disciplined ways of living give relief from pain whereas the best medical treatment failed. This is clear from the following case where acute back pain was cured by practicing yoga which involved a combination of physical exercise and systematic breathing.

Backache

Over three decades years ago I travelled in USA and Canada extensively by road by the luxury buses of the

Greyhound Company. I planned for two month's travel. Daily I covered about 500 miles. I travelled over ten thousand miles, enjoying the journey and the services. The tour covered some cities on the east and west coast.

On return to India I began feeling the impact of the long journey. I developed acute back ache which did not permit me to stand continuously even for twenty minutes. I tried allopathic treatment first. The physicians prescribed medicines which consisted of several tablets with varying dosages and for duration up to six-months. The medicines were mostly pain killers and gave only temporary relief. While in my home town I had morning walk covering a distance of 6 kms, daily. It gave me some relief.

Then I took ayurveda treatment but did not get lasting relief. Having tried these systems of treatment and finding lasting relief out of sight I explored alternatives. I had practiced yoga in my twenties and it helped me to maintain my weight and shape. But due to demands of the job and travelling I could not continue the exercises except occasionally.

Somehow it struck me that I should give yoga a trial for giving me relief. I decided to learn yoga lessons from a yoga master eight years ago. In 48 sessions I learnt essential yoga postures, known as asana, with rhythmic breathing. In two months results were experienced with relief. The training sessions lasted 90 minutes each. I practiced yoga regularly at home and chose a chain of postures practicing for 30minutes daily. These yoga postures involved stretching of limbs and muscles. With regular practice, in six months I got significant relief.

People learn yoga and with proper breathing and physical movements of various poses. They develop a healthy mind by doing meditation. Soon they find their body becoming flexible and of reduced weight. They get stamina and are able to stand any stress and strain without difficulty. This development does not take place overnight. Steady practice for a period of at least one year brings results. A side effect of these efforts is that clothing needs of these people who were in the heavy category feels the impact. The size of clothing and innerwear is reduced to half .They witness muscles being developed. Hypertension and body ache are eliminated. To one's surprise some find that even after twenty years their weight remains constant at 66 kgs for a height. of 178 cms. If some people can put in efforts steadily and shed off excess weight why not all in the category overweight try, strive and benefit.

The yoga postures were performed with proper breathing. Inhaling and exhaling were done appropriately for each posture. I devoted 30 minutes daily for practice in the morning and even now I continue to do this. The postures adopted were sarvangasana, chakrasana, bhujangasana, vajrasana, anjaneyasana and a few others. The details of these are given in any good yoga book. It is advisable to learn from a yoga teacher so that corrections if needed can be done and the postures perfected.

The test of the beneficial result was that I could undertake a road journey in the Himalayan region covering 1800 miles, walking in some places along narrow paths to places of worship located at heights varying from 10000 to 14000 feet. Later I could also stand in a mile long queue for worship at a temple in my home state on a very auspicious day for 8 hours. Fortunately the strenuous tasks did not leave any adverse impact except fatigue and pain for three days.

I have my yoga exercises daily even in my eightieth year. I do with ease and derive benefit. My weight is stable and it is well within limits for my height. I recommend yoga as a great remedy for those who suffer from back pain Vegetarian food is ideal for definite and quicker benefits.

Yoga is a great blessing we have inherited from ancient Indian heritage and wisdom. We are thankful to our ancestors. Yoga definitely helps to maintain mental and physical health. Yoga is conducive to happiness. If children are initiated to yoga early in life they will definitely benefit and can reduce the visits to the doctor and the incidence of illness.

Medical Journals publish tips for exercise and fitness, Body Mass Index calculator to keep track of how one is faring. In addition to the action mentioned earlier, some websites provide exercise tips that can help keep heart problems at bay. Of course, all the general medical websites propagate the benefits of exercise. Heart healthy exercise may be a key in warding off osteoarthritis, a "major cause of disability among adults over the age of 50."

Use of simple breathing exercises gives relief in stressful situations. Many people rely on exercise and participate in their favorite sports and games to dissipate piled up energy. Not all stress is bad e.g., stress in sports. Joining a sports team, even with co-workers can increase the enjoyment and relaxation level, and reduce tension. Games like golf, tennis, help people to relax. While counting factors contributing to stress count only one, such as calories, fat, cholesterol. More than one is confusing and discouraging, and thus doomed to failure.

Food

Maintaining health poses severe challenges. But eating right food is easy. Foods apparently simple, are easy to make, and have simple ingredients, are usually the best choices for right eating. They usually have a few ingredients and usually don't take long to cook. But it is difficult to make simple choices in the complex world of food stalls and restaurants?

But certain precautions are necessary for attaining success. We should abjure over eating. Gluttony is totally banned for such a person. A healthy body is essential for happiness. Extremes are bad. Food, exercise and recreation in moderate doses are good. There should be minimum spending of energy. Such a person is able to remove all sorrows. He enjoys complete tranquility of mind. He remains like a naked flame of a candle, well protected in a place where air cannot disturb, and where it doesn't flutter. His mind is full of optimism and anxiety to search for temporary pleasures does not arise. He is not disturbed by the greatest tragedy.

Whenever the mind runs away he brings it back for contemplation at the higher goal. Consistency of purpose is his secret of achievement. With faith in God obstacles vanish. Actions become more efficient. Grace is earned. With consistent thinking, disciplined effort and faith in the goal the direction is set. It works like a bullet. You cannot call it back.

The best way to choose between alternatives is to start with some research on the food. Reading labels of the products gives lot of information. . Most products today are trying to go "organic", "green", or "all natural" and that part of the label will usually be visible on the package. Reading the contents of the package is helpful for keeping our diet simple. As a general rule, if the ingredient list is long, it's probably not a simple food. A long list generally contains huge several additives and preservatives harmful to the person. The shorter the list, the better the food is for us. It will have the vitamins we need.

. Another general rule is that less food is best. Excessive sodium makes us thirsty; it builds up in our body and leads to an unhealthy heart. Excessive calories cause over weight and make us feel bloated. Sweets and potato chips occupy a place in any diet. There is nothing wrong in eating ice cream, unless one consumes it in excess. If you eat in moderation, your diet can be adequate and healthy. Even a modest reduction in food intake with excessive salt and fat together with regular physical activity can be beneficial.

Each food that you eat should come from one of the basic food groups. Sweets are in the basic pyramid. Fruits, vegetables, grains, are all important for a healthy diet. Exercise can complex or as simple as per your need. You could climb the stairs instead of the elevator, park your car a little further away in the parking lot while shopping and play in the park with kids.

Nutrition is one area of action for effective stress reduction. We eat daily at least thrice. Even the smallest of changes towards adopting a nutritious diet could bring about significant benefits. Stress can and does result from poor and insufficient nutrition; excessive use of intoxicants; negative emotions; lack of physical exercise; genetic factors; and improper body alignment.

We can reduce stress, prevent chronic diseases including depression and improve happiness through continuous mental fitness training. A complete nutritional approach, combined with proper fitness maintenance and stress management is very important. Exercise and physical fitness act as a buffer against stress. This ensures that stressful events have less negative impact on psychological and physical health. They switch over to nutritious food and vegetarian diet. Fruits and raw vegetables are introduced in the menu. Soon they find their weight again reduced by 5 kgs. The new food habits became a regular habit and changed lifestyle. They consume plenty of water and gave up carbonated drinks.

Cooking low fat meals is easy. You can live a healthy lifestyle with low fat consumption and exercise. Even at the age of 76 one measuring 5'-10" has a regulated weight of 65kgs. If one consumes junk food, smoke and does not exercise, one runs the risk of developing heart diseases in the thirties. According to medical studies, about 46.9 million Indians between 20 and 69 suffered from heart diseases by 2010 and half of them youngsters. Fast food has become the staple diet for majority of youngsters. They take soft drinks in place of water and spend hours sitting in front of computers. Sedentary lifestyle has made us vulnerable to cardiovascular diseases,"

Another general rule is that less food is best. Excessive sodium makes us thirsty; it builds up in our body and leads to an unhealthy heart. Excessive calories cause over weight and make us feel bloated. Sweets and potato chips occupy a place in any diet. There is nothing wrong in eating ice cream, unless one consumes it in excess. If you eat in moderation, your diet can be adequate and healthy.

Each food that you eat should come from one of the basic food groups. Sweets are in the basic pyramid. Fruits, vegetables, grains, are all important for a healthy diet. Exercise can complex or as simple as per your need. You could climb the stairs instead of the elevator, park your car a little further away in the parking lot while shopping and play in the park with kids.

The best way to choose between alternatives is to start with some research on the food. Reading labels of the products gives lot of information. . Most products today are trying to go "organic", "green", or "all natural" and that part of the label will usually be visible on the package. Reading the contents of the package is helpful for keeping our diet simple. As a general rule, if the ingredient list is long, it's probably not a simple food. A long list generally contains huge several additives and preservatives harmful to the person. The shorter the list, the better the food is for us. It will have the vitamins we need.

Maintaining health poses severe challenges. But eating right food is easy. Foods apparently simple, are easy to make, and have simple ingredients, are usually the best choices for right eating. They usually have a few ingredients and usually don't take long to cook. But it is difficult to make simple choices in the complex world of food stalls and restaurants?

Medicine without Side Effects

Human beings crave for good health, why the best health. Nobody wants to fall a prey to illness. Knowingly or unknowingly human beings adopt ways of living which they call life style. But this concept remains a style without life.

In fact there is no life in it. Many live on the assumption that eating and merry making constitute the essence of life. Many load their belly with food akin to filth and give free display to senses and sensuality.

Modern medicine, they think, provides cure for all illness and they console themselves saying that they can take shelter under the protective and secure wings of allopathy.Whether it is head, heart, hip or other body parts they feel confident medicine can cure their ailments. But medicine and doctors really do not cure. Wise medical practitioners who have great concern for the patient do not claim to cure illness. They give only relief. This is true also. In the name of cure quacks and charlatans recommend costly measures of treatment which often result in costly death. They are, with exceptions, fixing their eyes on the valet of the patient more than the values which their profession under the banner of Hippocrates professed. The wise among medical professionals believe and affirm that the cure is in the hands of a super power called God. They profess to be god-fearing men at least before the public.

Contrary to these champions of modern medicine we have millennium old method of treatment called Ayurveda. The profession of ayurvedic doctors is as over 4500 years old.

The architects of the ayurveda mode of treatment emphasized on the curative aspects of illness and went to the root of the problem. They discovered the link and interconnection between the mind, body and intellect. They also propagated the curative aspect of treatment attributed to the divine power and instilled spirituality in the treatment process. Leading *ayurvedic* hospitals installed a small temple of the God of medicine whom they called *Danwantari*. Before launching any treatment especially in severe cases, they worshipped *Danwantari* and then only proceeded. The patient also worshipped the deity. The sincerity of such professionals is seen in the correctness of the diagnosis, treatment, choice of medicines and in invoking the blessings of God.

They recommended a lifestyle with restrictions on food and daily routine. The objective was to improve the person's physical, emotional and spiritual components of lifestyle. *Ayurveda* imparted a healthy and steady lifestyle as part of the treatment process in a manner more convincing and beneficial than in any other branch of medicine and treatment.

. The central concept behind *Ayurveda* is to improve and ensure the individual's physical, emotional and spiritual equilibrium to attain self healing and increased longevity. Individuals suffering from emotional, mental or physical suffering, found the change over to a new lifestyle, beneficial by living an improved quality of life.

Ayurveda is the art of healing through the application of many natural methods including, Yoga, nutrition, herbs and massage. It integrates a holistic lifestyle choice, and provides for a natural life balance within the body through a combined approach. .

As a lifestyle preference *Ayurveda* necessitates various key points to consider. It requires a change in the dietary and physical activities apart from a complete change of one's daily schedule. It encourages the practice of waking up early, before sun-rise, to stimulate a positive phenomenon within the body attained through the peace and tranquility of nature. As a morning ritual, it recommends washing the face, mouth and, eyelids, followed by proper cleaning of the body through voluntary bowel movement. For many beginners, these practices may be a difficult transition to start with and achieve. However, through proper guidance, the body can be regulated to adapt to these new processes in a week.

The richness of the *ayurvedic* treatment is that it has no adverse side effects. The general health of the patient improves steadily. It eliminates pain .This cannot be effectively achieved by allopathic treatment. Pain in the joints, back ache, pain in the heels and elbows vanish with a course of treatment. The massage is done for an hour followed by steam bath in some cases. It is a wonderful experience. One feels a sense of wellbeing after the bath. During the treatment process the physician or his deputy lights a wick lamp and generally prays to God for the speedy and healthy recovery of the patient. This is a unique feature of *ayurveda*.

The tradition of ayurveda is very ancient and the cardinal principle observed by the physicians was that treatment and cure of the patient was the most important objective and remuneration for services was secondary and voluntary. Greed never dominated such treatment. No doubt medicines these days are expensive. But while charging the fee greed rarely gained the upper hand. The efficacy of *ayurveda* is now realized globally. India holds the key to cure by *ayurveda*. May the world benefit from the nectar of benefits flowing from such treatment linking herbs, nature and God.

4. Mental Health

Mind

Of all faculties of man, the mind is a remarkable one, a 10 billion dollar gift. It is said that if a machine is to be made to discharge the functions of the mind, it will cost at least $10 billion. Even then it will be a poor substitute for the mind, which travels faster than light. The moment you desire to be in a distant 5 billion light years away your mind takes you there. When we are blessed with such a precious gift, we have to ask ourselves whether we making the best use of it for the benefit of society and us. The answer is 'No'.

The choice of thoughts is decided by the intellect, which weighs pros and cons, discriminates and decides.

Intelligent men believe in living in the present. it is worth realizing that the present alone is within our control. The past is gone. We have no control over it. Today's present becomes tomorrow's past. Today's future becomes tomorrow present. So there is no past or future but only present. We must productively use the present moment before us and live in the present to get the best results from our efforts. We should not have preoccupations. . It does not mean we should not think of the future or learn from the past. We can learn lessons from the past to make improvements in the present, which will have impact on the future. We can plan for the future to devote our time usefully. Future is shaped by what we do in the present.

Desire originates in mind. If allowed to go unchecked it multiplies and creates agitations dissipating energy. If desires are not fulfilled anger arises and mental agitation follows. A satisfied desire leads to craving and soon greed overtakes us. All these depict the unbridled condition of the mind resulting in mental ill health and unhappiness. So we have to keep the mind steady and calm.

There is a beautiful example given in the Hindu scriptures, which makes us understand the role of the mind. The human body is compared to a chariot. The five senses are the horses and the reins represent the mind. The charioteer is the intellect. The occupant is God who is the witness to everything. For excellence in performance the senses have to be controlled. The mind does this under proper control and direction. For effective functioning it has to take orders from the intellect, which directs it without allowing going astray. When this happens harmoniously the chariot goes smoothly along the right royal road and to the destination.

Meditation

It is important for all and particularly for business executives to keep the mind steady and calm. Executives suffer stress, which is an undesirable experience. Everyone wants relief from stress. It clouds ones thinking, saps energy and health. The result is that a stress-affected person explodes out of bad temper. Some executives howl like wild beasts at subordinates and believe in the practice of animal control. This sets in motion a chain reaction and strained relationships in the organization. Progressive organizations will do well to include meditation as part of management techniques to attain human excellence and organizational harmony. They can control executive behavior molding it for organizational effectiveness. Laughter relaxes the mind and is the best medicine to relief stress. It costs nothing. Just like air, space, water, fire and earth it is free. The mind becomes fresh. Laugher tones up the system. Laughter therapy has come to be accepted as a useful technique for attaining mental health and harmony. Let us realize and fully utilize the great gift God has bestowed on us. Great achievers in any field are those who realized this potential and developed a universal mind. Let us move in that direction and inspire posterity. Thus we build a better world to live and enjoy.

The mind is a flow of thoughts occurring at random and sometimes with a purpose. It entertains negative and positive thoughts on different occasions. It has great potential for doing good and bad. Sometimes it is dull and at other times it is very active. It is restless and this aggravates if neglected. There is a case of a monkey to illustrate the seriousness of the restless mind. The monkey by itself is restless. It got intoxicated with liquor. In that condition a scorpion stung it. On the way it was seized by a devil. Now you can imagine its condition as a result of the cumulative impact of all these influences. So is the case with the human mind, which is uncared and nurtured with thoughts of anger and greed. We have sense organs for hearing, seeing, tasting, touching and smelling. Without the mind these organs are only matter. It is the mind behind the organs that makes them functional.

The seeds of wars are sown in the minds of men. This shows its destructive nature. The seeds of good deeds also originate in the mind and they form one's character and ultimately destiny. We have seen great scientists and leaders who applied their minds positively upholding noble and lofty ideals, ultimately bringing about great inventions, discoveries and achievements. We are not really attaining the potential of the mind. Except in rare cases, Hardly 0.1 per cent of it is utilized Human beings who have achieved high are those who have tapped the reservoir of energy within. Others fritter away such energy in ephemeral pleasures, entertainments, time wasting occupations, nonsensical conversation and gossip, which benefit none. The mind is a double-edged sword that can be use for killing an enemy or save a person. The great achievements of Nobel laureates reveal the positive and fruitful use of mind whereas those using destructive means reveal negative applications. Great men control the mind, conserve energy to benefit society and get a sense of fulfillment. They develop powers of concentration. Meditation helps to control the mind by focusing on a single idea or object on which thought flows without any break.

Your mental health will definitely help to promote your physical health. It inculcates discipline in you and with concentration you can complete your tasks efficiently. You have to preserve your physical health and for this regular exercise is needed. You can take a walk in the morning for 40 minutes after prayers. It can be a brisk walk, the speed depending on your age and agility. More beneficial results are obtained by changing the name of the Lord while walking.

This can be accompanied by rhythmic breathing. Deep inhalation and exhalation helps to tone up your system. You can inhale while covering the first two-steps and exhale while covering the next four footsteps. This strengthens the heart and ensures supply of more oxygen to all parts of the body. It can make you a man or woman with nerves of steel and muscles of iron.

Breathing is very important in ensuring mental and physical health. Soon after meditation in the morning you sit down on the floor, on a mat or some medium, with your legs crossed and pulled towards your thighs. You sit erect, look straight and inhale and exhale powerfully. When you inhale draw in maximum air inside. The belly will expand to the maximum like a balloon while inhaling. Then slowly exhale contracting the belly. When exhalation is complete the belly shrinks to the maximum creating a hollow externally. You are advised to breathe only through the nose. Repeat this gradually increasing it from 10 times to 20 or more according to time available. You should stop the process when you feel any sign of strain.

This pattern of breathing ensures increased supply of oxygen to all cells of the body and invigorates them. The exhalation dispels all impurities. You will feel considerable relief from stress and a sense of well-being. All through you will be focusing your attention on the midpoint between the eyebrows.

Later lie down on the floor on your back practically motionless keeping your feet slightly apart in a relaxed manner inhaling and exhaling deeply. This cycle can go up to 20 times or more depending on your stamina and time. If you practice this daily you will have a sense of physical well-being. You will find life enjoyable.

Always you meditate on Him and His glory. Chant His name as frequently as possible. With steady practice you will achieve calmness of mind and experience peace and tranquility. With such a frame of mind you can grasp any reading material fast and react peacefully and intelligently to the stimuli and the knowledge coming from external sources.

Change in schedule has to be made gradually. There should be a commitment to perform daily outdoor exercise. Changes in diet should take place slowly. Motivation is vital. No one should aim at sudden and substantial weight reduction. This should be in small variations. A kg a week is a realistic weight loss objective. We must review the position after six months, remembering this is helpful while checking your weight. Assessing how you're feeling and determining your increased energy level, participation in gymnastic activity and practice of yoga do lot of good. Meeting people who give encouragement to adopt a better life style is a beneficial experience.

Stress management should be a major concern for those seeking a healthy lifestyle. A commitment to live a healthier lifestyle is a desirable objective. Stress management is not only an urgent need in today's hectic lifestyle, but an important factor in both physical and mental health. Stress is more the result of one's lifestyle. Eliminating stress producing factors and/or gaining healthy insight on how to alleviate stress effectively is the best thing for an individual to do for himself. People who have acquired spiritual strength are in a far better position to withstand stress compared to those who are not so .They are calm and never get rattled by adverse circumstances.

To be happy one will find it helpful to meditate on the Ultimate Reality. This means stretching one's mind to the farthest. One can be happy or unhappy at the mental level, can have comfort or discomfort at the body level and have peace or disturbance at the intellectual level. Physical exercises have lot to do with mental and psychic development. Inhalation, exhalation, holding breath, control of diet and food ensure purity of mind and intellect. Every successful human being practices self-control. Such persons protect themselves from distractions. They adopt different ways of economizing energy and preventing dissipation of mental energy. This is Royal wisdom or Royal secret. It is the Royal science of living.

It is the most effective purifier. The mind and intellect have no source of disturbance. Mankind should move to a higher plane of consciousness. There should not be any vacillation. All living beings have to be looked with reverence and respect. This needs consistency of effort. Meditation enables us to turn the attention of the mind and intellect in a specific angle. It demands total surrender to the Lord. Having known and become that state which is a permanent experience one never returns to the lower nature. One should aim to be happy and contented. Meditation is helpful and the body has to be maintained in good health. This is achieved through a series of physical exercises combining breathing.

Setting apart some time daily in the morning preferably for meditation brings great benefit ensuring a calm mind. Choose a quiet place. Sit erect, close your eyes and breathe normally after deep inhaling and exhaling a few times. Inhale and fill the lungs with air. Observe moderation in eating and food habits and sleep. . The place chosen should be clean and peaceful. This can be inside the home, outside in the open visualizing a mountain or an ocean or the Sun. Bring the flow of thoughts to that object which you have firmly fixed in your mind. Think about the glory of that object. Ignore if all sorts of thoughts interfere and disturb your thought flow in the desired direction. In course of time and with steady practices this will be all right.

The unique nature of man is that he alone has the faculty of discrimination. He alone is endowed with the capacity to realize the Ultimate truth. which is the changeless knowledge .By constant practice we find the complete merger of the principle with the individual, merging into one and this enables solutions to all problems of the world? Thus is beautifully stated in the Shanthi Mantra of the Hindus .This when translated says, "Let us both be protected. Let both of us enjoy together. Let what is given to us become glorious. Let there be no hatred. O Peace. Peace, Peace". Humans face three types of sorrow. The first one is natural calamities. The second one is from external objects and the third one from within which has spiritual orientation.

Mind conquered is available and this helps to lift you by yourself. It is a great friend. It no more entertains endless desires. Such a person is extremely contented He is unshaken. He has an integrated mind. To such a man, in terms of attitude, clay and a brick of gold are the same. His wealth is bliss. He practices meditation seeking the state of pure happiness.

Power of thoughts is the greatest inner wealth. He develops moral and ethical values all positive values. non-hatred sympathy. and friendship. He is totally unselfish and has no ego. He never complains. He does not distribute sorrow but sows happiness. He is cheerful under all conditions and firm in his convictions with mind and intellect in total surrender to Him. Preserving intellectual and mental vitality is the secret of achievement of such men. The world doesn't fear them.

The qualities of joy, envy, sorrow are born out of body consciousness. Having gone beyond these qualities properties of the body no longer affects him. Death, old age and sorrow do not affect him He enjoys luminosity and engages in endless series of activity. There are no selfish desires since all activities are for benefit of mankind. He is firmly set like a lighthouse on a rock. He is equal to praise or blame. love and hatred, jeers and cheers, joy and sorrow, and friend and foe. This is the greatest secret of sciences. Wisdom demands assimilation and absorption so that every thought will have a golden view. We can enrich our life by giving up the anxieties to enjoy the fruits of action.

When you sit up for meditation several obstacles will arise. Mind will wander. Unpleasant thoughts will interfere with meditation. You know the mind is a monkey. It is very difficult to tame it. But this does not mean that you should not try. Every attempt to bringing back the mind to the object of meditation is a step forward. Think of the vast universe, the ocean, and the mountain and visualize them while meditating. Even if you slip you will reach one stretch of sea from another. You will reach one star from another. So the course will not be deflected though the point of concentration will shift for a while. There are situations when one is gripped by depression and despondency. Take for example the plight of a monkey, which by itself is restless, gets dead drunk, is bitten by a scorpion and is possessed of a ghost. We should not succumb to such a situation.

. **Conquer Boredom**

Many people feel and often complain of severe boredom in their life. They lament that this is a trap from which they are unable to escape and thus are resigned to their fate. In fact it is not really so. Boredom is one's own creation. It can be totally eliminated. Let us explore how this is done with an understanding of the nature of boredom.

When does one say he is facing boredom? This happens when one finds time is hanging on his neck and is unable to pass on usefully. Every minute is a prolonged period as if it were several hours of lethargic existence. The victim feels he is doing nothing. Out of disgust he goes on munching something in between meals or tries various alternatives to get rid of boredom. Some time is spent in TV watching, phoning up friends, reading light novels, and doing some domestic work. Still there is lot of time left to be spent and time does not move. His mind is clogged not knowing what to do. Let us consider a few examples.

Sometimes in our attempt to overcome boredom we go out to witness some art performance or music recital, but even then after a few minutes we experience boredom. We attend a drama. One of the scenes involves two persons entering into a dialogue which is monotonous and never ending. In another case a person attends a conference. One of the speakers goes at a tangent, exceeds his time limit, and talks utter nonsense. The audience is bored. They don't know how to get over the situation. They wait for someone to break open and flush out the bore.

The musical bore was packed off by cooperative effort. Many from the audience sent slips of paper with title of a piece which reached the musician. He thought that they were asking for some popular song to be sung and looked cheerful. But this was short-lived when he opened the slips only to find that all of them unanimously suggested that he sang the concluding song which normally took one minute and thus closed the recital. In the case of the boring dialogue the bore was banished by a guest who went right up to the stage, shook hands congratulating the artiste on his performance and then politely telling him the audience would have a full-length demonstration of his skills some other day.

The conference bore was handled by a senior bold dashing member who first sent a polite reminder that time was running out. But when there was no end to his frontal attack he walked up to the stage and told him in harsh words that he was talking irrelevant and should stop. The speaker relented and left.

These are cases where the source of boredom is external and some drastic measures are called for. But when the boredom is within the individual and when time is not moving fast, it crawls at snail's pace. What is the alternative open to such a person? It is helpful to have hobbies which use creativity of the mind.

Painting, listening to good music, writing, reading books of great interest and enlightenment, spending time with family particularly grand children, playing games with members of the family attending seminars and lectures etc. are some of the ways by which boredom can be eliminated. The essence is that the mind should be fully occupied. Then there will be no awareness of time and you will enjoy the activity undertaken.

Boredom is essentially one's own creation. It is a condition of the mind .To overcomes this we have to engage the mind in useful activities. It is possible to attain this by steady practice.

It is possible to be happy and remain without an agitated mind by changing our attitude towards the environment, goods and services. God has given us everything as a gift. We are only His trustees. The world has enough to meet our needs but not our greed. Can't we curtail our greed?

5. Facing Misfortunes

Many of us some time or other have experienced misfortunes. We have felt that the whole world is going against us and we are thrown into the sea of misery. This happens when the gap between expectation and fulfillment is very wide. Sudden illness, untimely death of a close relative, unexpected failure in an examination, loss in business due to market collapse are some examples of this painful feeling which creates mental unrest and agony and sets in motion a chain of misery. We strongly feel this when we suffer a lot when others succeed and are happy. They accomplish effortlessly great tasks whereas we have to slog and struggle. What we fail to achieve with a ton of energy others attain with an ounce of effort. It is not merely the quality of effort but something beyond. The environment is favorable to the person who puts in least effort and hostile for the other. The loss of energy, time and money in some cases is considerable. It becomes difficult to reconcile with the situation. The return on effort is very poor. The victim indulges in a game of cursing himself. Some others find fault with others. Students who fail in the examination despite hard work blame others. Sometimes they consider life not worth living, feel disgusted and believe that everything is lost. This causes poor and strained relationships within the family and circle of friends. A marriage, which started with great hopes, soon crash-lands and the first tendency is to blame luck or misfortune. A feeling of acute depression sets in. The victim becomes lonely unable to face friends and colleagues. A feeling of utter helplessness dominates and the victim is unable to come out of the trap.

But there is a bright side to this problem of helplessness. We also find persons who too face very adverse situations but overcome them without any scar on their minds. Let us take one example. A pious, religious businessman having implicit faith in God runs a business, which he started with a small capital. It grew fast and he became a leading exporter winning national awards for excellence in export performance Profits soared. He continued to have faith in God and help people as he used to do before. The demand for his products could not be met. It was so high that foreign buyers engaged chartered vessels for acquiring huge quantities from his area of operations. He maintained quality and earned a reputation for ethical business dealings. So his brand earned a premium. In view of the growing demand, often unfulfilled, he installed large additional processing capacity with borrowed funds. His factory became the biggest one in Asia. When production was at its peak and orders were flowing he built up stocks expecting them to be shipped within a month The trade practice was that the buyer's agents issued purchase orders based on which bank financed for processing goods. Letters of credit were opened later and they arrived just before shipment.

Business was going on smoothly. All in a sudden the international oil crisis emerged. The world economic environment turned hostile and the demand for his products slumped. His was a 100% export oriented industry and the entire production was for the foreign markets. The buyers recast priorities and cancelled all orders. He had stocks of $10 million. It could not be sold in any other market let alone domestic market. Even at one twentieth of the price there were no takers. The goods became dead stock. They had to be dumped in the sea. Bankers pressed for clearing huge liability. Interest and principal mounted sky high.

Many firms in the industry suffered the same fate. The loss varied depending on the size of the firm. But the directors of the company maintained their calm and were never agitated. They could not continue business for a long time. They had high business ethics and continued to have full faith in God. This was seen visibly in all their dealings with others and with the bankers. Wisdom prompted them to prepare a concrete proposal to the bankers for settling the liabilities. They willingly sold most of the assets and started clearing the liabilities. The bankers realizing their honest dealings and intentions gave substantial concessions in interest arrears. This helped to reduce the liability. Ultimately they cleared off the entire liability. It took seven years, no doubt.

This is a genuine and interesting case of one facing misfortune, living with it gracefully and finally overcoming it. The clear conscience and the faith in God helped a lot to maintain calm and think clearly and positively about what needed to be done to come out of the situation. They had the courage to bury the business when they found that was the best option possible and a wise one in such circumstances.

Lessons from such cases give us the strength and courage to face situations and overcome the worst instances of misfortune. We have to take them in our stride remaining unruffled. When we are not avaricious, when we observe high degree of business ethics, and deal with employees and others with fairness and equity we will have the grace of the Almighty and that helps us to overcome this difficulty.

6. Depression

Can we get rid of worry or stop worrying? Yes it is definitely possible. How? The first prerequisite for attacking worry and to overcome the problem is to have firm determination to improve and try evolving a worry free life. The various steps to be followed are given below:

Identify the problem worrying the person. Isolate it and ask questions to find answers. Is it non-attainment of anything considered desirable? Is it about the health or well being of a person? Is it lack of finance for commanding anything? Is it damage of any material/ equipment considered precious?

Isolate the person, event, or thing from you. If it is a person, ask what worries him. How are you concerned with him? Clearly think and determine whether it is your responsibility in any way. If there is no one else to remove his worry why should you take it over? If action is to be taken by him/others, advise him/them. Action arising from a spirit of service and not attachment based on ignorance is the weapon to deal with worry. Detachment is made possible by de-linking the mind from the object or person. While you may have a duty to see that he is in worry free state, you should not be craving for the result. Craving brings mental uneasiness.

Realize that worrying does not solve the problem. Solution is purely through an intellectual process determining in a sequence a series of steps to be taken by you. This may/may not need financial help. Break the problem into simple parts and with a detached view take one by one for analysis and the solution will emerge. This clear intellectual process requires a calm mind, which in turn requires meditation. Continued meditation helps to get rid of worries by revealing the line of action needed to eliminate worry.

The same is applicable to things and finance. Financial worry almost kills a person. With meditation, a clear mind and intellect is obtained. With these tools problems can be dissected and with the sword of non-attachment solution found. Ask yourself what action is necessary. Do not postpone action. Prompt action dissolves worry quickly.

You can insulate your mind against worry. This is by mentally chanting the name of the Lord, which does not allow any disturbing thought to enter. It is like placing a leaf inside a pot full of water. This helps spillage and preserves the water inside. It absorbs all shocks due to movements. Thus calmness of mind is ensured. Worry free living can be experienced. Any work can be done simultaneously with chanting the Lord's name since Over 99% of the mental capacity is available for work, which can be done with greater efficiency.

Many patients fall a prey to mental illness called anxiety and depression. Their mood and enthusiasm dampen entering a trough of despondency from which they can't escape. The remedy for depression depends on attitude change and this is more effective than medicines and tranquilizers. Depression is a state of mind. The mind is seized by dark thoughts which appear like a trap imprisoning the intellect. The individual is unable to think through and find a way out. He feels a high sense of insecurity. Some burst into tears thus spreading the misery to others.

Such individuals feel they are not loved and not wanted by anyone. They in disgust resign themselves into a state of utter helplessness and succumb to a strong feeling of disappointment murmuring that Life did not shape according to their plan. They always remain pessimistic, blaming the environment for all sad events. They don't care to analyze their experiences. Nor do they try to find out the basic cause for the present state of affairs. They brood over their rudderless existence and the feeling strengthens that life is going out of control and everything is going to crash-land. Anxiety eats away our energy. Medicines are only temporary and partial solution to the problem which is of one's own making.

Materialistic things can interfere with our daily relationship with the Lord. If one spends too much time showing off ones wealth and acquisitions one can lose sight of what's important: ones relationship with the divine power. Materialistic things can interfere with our daily union with God. Remember that without that Supreme Power called God, we wouldn't have any of those essential items which we take for granted. If we brood over why we don't live in a palatial luxurious mansion, or why we drive a bucket on wheels, rather than a BMW we make ourselves miserable and live in continued depression. The amount of money we spend on material things takes us away from spiritual life.

Our desire for more and more materialistic things and comforts goes unabated.
Men with simple life styles feel guilty of spending lavishly when they see people around struggling to eat and keep a roof over their heads. They don't realize that, Nature or Mother Earth has provided us the basics, such as food and clothing.

We need a little more of spirituality, a little less of sensuality and a new perspective on the material things of this world. We brought nothing into this world, and it is certain we can't take out even a needle.

Most people cannot escape stress inducing stimuli, but must learn to cope constructively. Exercise plays a key role in keeping a healthy mind by releasing chemicals, improving circulation throughout the body and to the brain, and by reducing stress related hormones. Meditation, reading, listening to music, or anything else that diverts the mind from negativity is valuable as well. Yoga is very effective to accomplish both exercise and meditation. The most basic yoga routines include specific exercises that encourage proper digestion.

Certain herbal remedies also help to reduce stress and to promote relaxation. They are often available as combinations and sold in bulk, pill form. It is becoming increasingly easy and affordable to make use of these natural stress solutions, especially when compared to their pharmaceutical counterparts which are usually expensive, and may have serious health implications.

The same idea remains true for digestive remedies. Pharmaceutical digestive medicines are generally created to alleviate symptoms, but do not necessarily serve to establish balance. Antacids, for instance, neutralize stomach acids which are needed to break down food properly. This extinguishes the painful symptoms of improper digestion, but may advance the severity of the condition by discouraging adequate nourishment. Other symptomatic medications such as pain relievers, antibiotics, and anti-inflammatory drugs destroy the body's enzymes.

Remember the most essential things in life air, water, space, fire are free. If any agency were to charge for these services or facilities it will come to an enormous amount. But for the Supreme Power which made this available to us we save so much money and use it for other purposes. Intelligence has to be used with discrimination and man has to learn to be contented. He has to develop an attitude of working for the joy of work. Of course one should earn and get remuneration for the work done. But wealth and its acquisition have to be based on righteousness. Otherwise greed will dominate and engulf humanity. The recent recession is an example of the global dimensions of the calamity resulting from greed, yes, unbridled greed. Let us not repeat such an occurrence. In that attitude and state of mind there will be no anxiety and depression.

7. Marital Conflict

As civilization advances and material progress takes place marital conflicts and divorce cases are increasing. Family harmony, the cornerstone of happiness in ancient times, is vanishing in many cases to an alarming degree. Marital conflicts arise mostly from temperamental differences. Initial neglect of these differences and indifference towards finding solutions blow them up beyond control. They result in open and violent eruption of differences and in some cases divorce. No society considers increasing tendency towards divorces as a healthy development. But are society and its constituents serous about reversing this trend? Can we reverse this trend or reduce its intensity and magnitude?

Marriage legally brings together man and woman, persons from different families with differing background, ways of living and perhaps culture. Rarely do we have a case of an ideal marriage. The temperament of one of the partners may be sweet and the other short or abrasive. There may be conflict of interests and priorities. Their intellectual attainments may be unequal and these sometimes reveal a wide gap between the two personalities.

The trouble starts when one has a positive attitude towards life, events and actions whereas the other displays a negative attitude. Unless efforts are made to develop positive attitudes by the one lacking them, the gap widens. One may say the other person having positive attitudes has to narrow the gap by cultivating negative attitudes towards achieving parity. But this is an undesirable solution wrought with disastrous consequences. It can never be called an adjustment or remedy.

Another cause of disharmony is mutual suspicion. In most cases the suspicion may be baseless and can be removed by frank discussion. If suspicion continues a situation arises that there is no openness in the family and one feels like a thief in one's own home. Children are also affected and they learn negative tendencies from such parents engaging in conflicts.

There are cases of economic independence where one of the partners asserts too much giving rise to conflicts which are not resolved. There is a power struggle and one dominates the other because of a feeling of independence, superiority or dominance. Nagging is another sad phenomenon. There is reluctance to move together while making social calls.

The impact of this obsession is transmitted to friends and relatives while they visit or who are visited out of compulsion. There is no openness in conversation and feelings are suppressed. Discussions turn into arguments and emotions come into play with a final flare up and outburst. Both parties feel great discomfort and agony in that situation and it is sheer luck if one of them walks out of the situation to allow tempers to cool.

In all cases the conflict arises due to both parties losing sight of the common goal of family harmony and happiness. The situation is ignited when differences are ignored at the initial stage and when the parties go on harping on differences. They show intolerance, disregard reason and emotions of the other. The partners lack understanding and are forgetful of the family as one unit and its cohesiveness.

To overcome the situation of marital conflicts and to prevent divorces the parties involved can set family management objectives where harmony and happiness are given prime concern. Differences should not be allowed to reach a point of ignition. Discussions are advisable and arguments should be avoided. There should be attempts to discuss and solve differences amicably. When there is threat of discussion developing into argument one of the parties can leave the scene for some time or change the topic. This will extinguish the fire in the argument and help to restore normalcy. Efforts can be made by developing positive attitudes by the one now having negative ones. To the extent this succeeds the progress towards harmony will be steady and attainable.

After series of earnest attempts if the situation does not improve, as a last resort, divorce may be considered. When divorce takes place, the persons can remain as friends without animosity just as in the case of any other good friend. It devolves on each citizen as a responsible member of society to avoid marital conflict and divorce and help others to solve differences without conflict. This is possible in most cases. Marriage is a sacred institution. The family is the smallest administrative unit. Every citizen has to strive hard to preserve the sanctity of these time honored institutions.

8. Other intangibles

Humor

Laughter is important for happiness. It melts fog from man's face. For ages all the religions, preachers and Masters have talked about happiness and how to achieve it. Religions have focused on renunciation and elimination of desire. However, one can find happiness in this life in this world. Desire is an engine of material progress. If suppressed or removed it becomes sorrow. If sublimated it reveals happiness.

Humor can impart great nourishment to you in everyday life? It is beneficial to start the day with a beaming smile at yourself looking at the mirror followed by a few minutes of giggling laughter. Watching funny movies, reading articles on humor and cracking jokes with children can take you to higher level of health and wellbeing.

Loud laughter can increase heart rate, increase oxygen supply to the human system and strengthen the immune mechanism. It increases the level of immunoglobulin in the saliva. This helps the body to fight off infection e.g., the common cold. . Humor is contagious, and you can make many others laugh and boost your importance and self esteem.

`Humor helps to change man's mood in a very short time. It washes off anger. .Parents find humor a handy tool to discipline a mischievous child .Laughing stimulates the brain, and helps to acquire and store more information rendering humor an effective aid to studies.

People with a great sense of humor are able to laugh at themselves. They very rarely experience depression and anxiety. They see the world in a different perspective, because of their sense of humor. Smiling and laughter change negative emotions into positive ones. They help us feel better about ourselves. ` The medical profession recommends laughing as a therapy.

On an average children laugh over 200 times a day in contrast the adult has a poor score. Babies start smiling in a month soon after birth, and laughing soon after. And once they start, they keep doing it-over and over as they go through early childhood. The average adult laughs much less. It is less than 20 times per day. It is sad to note adults lose all sense of humor as they grow up. We don't realize that humor can make us healthier.

Laughing helps to lower blood pressure, burn calories, activates our internal organs. and almost the whole body. It reduces stress levels, ensuring calmness. Humor helps a person to overcome feelings of anxiety resulting from isolation. It is integral to peace of mind. In crises situations, humor gives hope. Spontaneous humor relieves tension and overcomes fear and anxiety during crisis. `

With illness and even death occurring, hospitals have come to believe that even a small dose of laughter can do lot of good for others apart from the patients! However there are safeguards to be taken while trying to be humorous. We must ensure appropriateness of humor to the occasion. Otherwise, humor can be harmful. Look at the following example. A person is asked to interview selected customers. He is asked to prepare a questionnaire which contains several questions. One question is," Are you married". The second question is "if yes, ask how many children"

Instead of reading and understanding the questions and the questionnaire the interviewer asks: "Are you married"

The customer answers, "No".

The interviewer asks, "How many children"

Though the answer can be interpreted as humorous the occasion is inappropriate since the customer, if touchy and sensitive can react violently defeating the purpose of the interview.

Radiate laughter all around. trying to get people to laugh with you. You may not always succeed. Some people are determined to be morose and miserable. But you could try to make them cheerful. Make them laugh with humorous anecdotes. Laughter helps you to improve your attitude.

Change in attitude makes you look at the world with a different perspective and enjoy life.

We come across several types of humor and humorists. A quick analysis of their contribution and characteristics bring them in some of the categories. Of the many three are listed above in the quote. It will be useful and interesting to examine each category with examples.

Let us take up the person who has an inventory of wit. He makes fun of others. To illustrate: we have the example of a person who sings and a handful of friends who are the listeners forming part of the audience.

One among the audience remarks: "Mr. Henry is a happy man. He always sings. He has no worries."

Mr. James supplements this comment. "Yes, quite true, when he sings all the worries go to others- the listeners. He thus becomes happy."

Then we take up the case of a satirist. He makes fun of the world. An example follows:

Orator: The credit for the achievement of keeping people poor in some countries goes to the politicians who have become power seekers, power brokers and power mongers.

Now follows the third category of people who ignite laughter. They're humorists in the real sense. They make fun of themselves. This is amplified below with an example.

The scene is with reference to a portrait of eminent academicians on the wall in the College.

Professor: One day I will also be hanging here.

This person makes fun at his own expense.

Humor does not have malice. It triggers laughter, stretches and relaxes all muscles in the face and the stomach. It entertains and enlarges the circle of friends. It is a trait worth developing.

Music

There is a saying that a man has no music in him is either God or beast. Every man loves and appreciates music, which has no boundaries. It appeals to all. Each country has music suited to its genius. It is admitted that music is soothing to the ears and the mind. It lifts one to a higher plane of mental existence. It enervates. It dissolves worries. It is used as a therapy to treat and cure illness. Each country has made its contribution to the development of music.

It is something, which comes out of inspiration. If we take for example Indian classical music we find a rich variety. It has melody appealing to the ears and theme to vibrate the heart. It has divinity because it is sung in praise of God in some form describing His glory. It is inspirational. Great musicians like Saint Thyagaraja devoted their entire lifetime for singing the glory of God through composing several thousand songs. These songs have simple philosophy and rich meaning easily understandable to the ordinary folk. They inspire millions of people who have the ears for melody and who can understand the basics of music. The philosophical content in the songs guide man for improving his nature and hasten the progress towards salvation.

Music uplifts the mind. It creates a unique sensation. Apart from enjoyment arising from the melody, the involvement of the listener produces sensations within. Man feels he is taken to a higher plane of mental existence, which helps to establish communion with the Almighty because of the philosophical meaning of the verses. The compositions are spontaneous creations arising from inspiration. They are the products of a mind, which derives happiness in singing. The flow of thoughts is purely divine in praise of God. The singer or composer establishes communion with the Almighty and this is seen in the content and melody of the song. He is pouring out his heart in full love and total surrender to the Almighty. It has the highest philosophy. Sometimes the composer laments that in spite of constantly singing the glory of Him he has not been blessed with the presence of God. It contains appeal to Him to bestow mercy on him. It shows his eagerness to be with him.

The singer appeals to Him to be considerate. The spiritual content of the song is seen without any adulteration of worldly desires and wants. The songs with their melody and spiritual content are a dependable medicine to patients suffering from chronic diseases. There are hospitals administering music as therapy to patients. In the case of terminal illness this is reported to work wonders. Pain is reduced. Patients become cheerful. They show a sense of relief and find pain less excruciating. The devotional content of the songs helps them to take to their illness and the inevitability of death calmly. These composers did not have any expectations of monetary reward when they sang. Their only aim was self-fulfillment and to benefit others. They did not fall a victim to the temptations of wealth and honor despite their poverty and trying circumstances.

. The musical notes when sung with variations present a very enjoyable feeling and the mind is swayed in great joy. This takes one to a contemplative mood from which no one wants to return.

This does not mean all forms of music have the same beneficial effect on others. In the name of music some practice strenuously what they call music, which turns out to be cacophony. It gives the feeling that they are producing jarring noise, which they alone enjoy. This is often done to earn name and fame but the result is an inflammable lethal dose of boredom to the audience. To illustrate, we give the reaction of a listener exposed to listening to music. Someone pointed out that Mr. was a happy man. He always sings and he has no worries. The listener said, "Yes. Very true. When he sings all worries go to others. Their worry is that they have to listen."

Prayer

Man often wonders why he should have faith in God. Sometimes he thinks God is nonexistent. According to many the living philosophy is gross materialism. They believe human birth is without purpose and is just accidental. It is foolish to believe in God as a super power guiding our destinies. It only weakens our personality making us poor achievers. There are others who believe in the existence of God. They believe God is an entity sitting far above in the sky beyond the clouds dispensing judgments over us. There are others who believe God is not an entity. It is spirit, the supreme consciousness. It is the cause of everything we see in this universe. Our aim is not to conduct any research into this interesting subject. As utilitarian's or rationalists, though not saints or sages, we can examine the expression God and try to understand whether we can benefit by believing or otherwise.

Our birth as a human being has given us an advantage over animals and other forms of life. While they have the same biological needs as man, we have the faculty of discrimination, which the animals and other forms of life do not have. It is this quality which makes man a unique being. It is up to him to make the best use of this faculty or engage in futile discussions. Being intelligent beings we would like to use our faculties with a purpose and for useful activities.

Let us examine our role. In this universe consisting of billions of galaxies with billions of stars and trillions of planets we live in one planet called the earth. Our sun, the source of all energy and light is only one of the trillions of stars in the galactic system. It is one of the billions of stars in the Milky Way galaxy, which is its home as well as ours. The Milky Way galaxy consists of 600 billion planets. Even after millions of years we have not developed the means of knowing whether there is any earth like planet among them supporting life in any form or as we have experienced. In this vast universe, which is ever expanding, we are suspended like a tiny ball in space with many billions of objects moving around us. So any time we are susceptible to collide with asteroids and big meteors like the one, which hit Arizona 65 billion years ago wiping out the largest living creatures the dinosaurs.

In this vast universe where is man? He is not even a tiny speck. He has intelligence but he has no knowledge of existence of life in any other planet. The earth moves at a speed of over 1300 miles per hour around the sun. Millions of asteroids are traveling in the path between the sun and earth. We have knowledge of only 10% of them but 90% remains outside our field of knowledge. There is every possibility of a hit from an asteroid. Can man do anything to prevent this? Can science and technology design a foolproof system to overcome this? Floods, melting of arctic ice, earthquakes, tsunami and the like occur every year. These cause severe damage to life and property. Can man do anything to prevent them? There are dangers from men around us, countries around us and from animals .We can prevent them to a limited extent. But can we always be safe. There are so many such cases where our precarious existence is brought to our mind often.

We all know there is some superior power than man, which has created this universe. You may call it Nature or anything. But what is the cause of the Nature. Scientists say it is energy, which is all pervading. From energy matter is created and matter disintegrates into energy. Energy is something scientist can determine. But how is energy caused. If we go to the root of all these phenomena we arrive at one thing, which is the basic cause. That is what we call God. It has no beginning or end. It is clearly seen from the experience of great Indian sages who retired to the deep forests and the Himalayas and searched for the truth with the only tool of self-introspection open to them. They sharpened their mind by meditation, contemplation and singleness of purpose and went in pursuit of the

Ultimate Reality. They have found an answer. This answer has come in the form of Vedas and Upanishads. That is God at the root of all material things we can imagine. Max Mueller the great German Philosopher said, "If there is one place on this planet where the human mind has probed into the problems of mankind and found lasting solutions I would point my finger at India". This is the affirmation of great men. The ultimate cause is God or Brahman, which is the expression, used by great sages of India. It is the spirit. It is supreme consciousness. It is other than the body, mind and intellect. Every living being has the spark of divinity within forming part of the whole. It is just like the space inside a pot becoming one with the space outside when the pot is broken.

There is a supreme power beyond our materialistic physical world. The cause for it is given in Hinduism, which permits application of the most powerful intellect. Hinduism gives a convincing explanation of what God is and how to realize it. For all problems of mankind, which are fundamental to man, the answer lies in Hinduism. The same quest which a scientist striving towards the Nobel prize if done in the pursuit of the knowledge of the absolute reality, making sacrifices as part of the discipline, he will definitely arrive at the conclusion that there is God and it is universal consciousness, the Supreme Consciousness. This according to Hinduism is Brahman, which can be understood only by some indications and not by definition. It can never be defined for definition limits its omniscience.

To explain that God exists and is without beginning and end, the example of a spider and the cobweb is narrated. The spider creates its cobweb from its saliva, which after some time goes to it. Similarly the universe originated in Brahman, exists in Brahman and goes back into it. The universe has come from the spirit i.e., the universal consciousness All matter originated from the five elements space, air, fire, water and earth Even materially speaking we have to believe in a great power called God. It is not separate from us. It is the universal consciousness. Man faces three categories of dangers .One is within man, lack of spiritual strength, sorrow, illness and restlessness. The second one is external to man i.e., wars, and conflicts, and wild animals. The third one is natural calamities: floods, earthquakes, and tsunami, tornados, collision with asteroids etc. These cannot be eliminated or avoided. In the case of the last one our strength is too inadequate and the only alternative open to us is Prayer, which is reassuring our faith in God, the supreme power that is implored to save us. The greater the intensity with which we pray the more is the likelihood of relief. If no relief comes we have the strength to accept the outcome as divine summons. We all know how the entire humanity prayed when the astronauts in Apollo XIII mission faced a crisis while re-entry, a threat to their lives, over which we could do nothing except pray. The collective prayers of the entire humanity including those in churches and other religious institutions were answered by some supreme power and that brought back the astronauts safely. So we feel happy in believing in God and let us maintain this happiness forever.

Human life is a precious gift of God. In the course of existence we experience pleasure and pain, happiness and sorrow. Earthly people want pleasure without pain but this cannot always continue. There is a way to attain a state of mind free form the influence of pain and sorrow. For those who are prepared to make sacrifices, practice with great determination and concentration this is attainable. Ordinary mortals, who desire to be free from sorrow or to minimize it, will find prayer is the most important means.

Prayer is addressed to God. In their vision and wisdom our ancestors always thought of the welfare of the entire humanity. Their vision brought forth verses which have eternal relevance and significant for the entire mankind.

Even for those busy with mundane things of life they had only love and composed verses to bring them relief from ordinary causes of sorrow and pain. Even those who want happiness without sorrow the verses enable them to march towards spiritual progress. Of course right attitude definitely helps to ward off sorrow and enables one to attain a state beyond happiness and sorrow or pain and pleasure. This is called bliss.

Knowing sorrow persists; the sages of wisdom in their vision discovered the root causes of sorrow and weaved verses covering all aspects of sorrow. In the normal course it is impossible to eliminate sorrow permanently. Man's efforts have their limitations. So prayer is only answer. We will consider here one such verse and its contents.

"Runa rogadhi daridrya papa kshutha apamruthyuvaha
Bhaya krodha manaklesha nasyanthu mama sarvadha"

This verse depicts all types of sorrow. These are beautifully classified under nine heads. The sources of sorrows are anger, debt, disease, decay, fear, poverty, premature death, sin and worry. The prayer is addressed to the Almighty to relieve one from all sorrows.

All sorrows are listed in the nine categories. Anger is an unpleasant feeling of anguish. Debt creates an obligation and anxiety if it exceeds repaying capacity. Disease produces a feeling of anxiety and restlessness of mind. Decay of the body causes concern. Fear of anything is a source of sorrow till we overcome it. Poverty deprives us of essentials to existence and is thus sorrowful. Premature death brings sorrow when are threatened. Sin gives a feeling of sorrow or regret. Worry is a source of sorrow.

We must make our own efforts to get rid of these aspects of sorrow. But to gain the strength to ward off these sources of sorrow we pray and chant the mantra listing these nine categories. We pray to God to give us the wisdom to take timely action to ward of these undesirable influences. It is right thinking that enables us to act rightly in accordance with tested wisdom. So the prayer is addressed to the Almighty to purify our thoughts. By constant chanting of the mantra we are attuned to the contents and are in a better frame of mind to face the world. May there be peace and happiness to all

Noble Thoughts

Everything originates from thoughts. An idea takes shape from thoughts. After scrutiny and deliberation it becomes an act. When several acts take place a character is formed. In the long run one's destiny evolves from such a character. That is the power of thought.

It is up to us to make a thought noble or otherwise. Noble thoughts are those which ensure welfare of society and of oneself. They result in noble acts and constant performance of noble acts makes a noble character. Such an individual is an asset to society. Great leaders in all walks of life have made significant contributions. They have always entertained noble thoughts and through noble acts achieved greatness for the country and for themselves.

We benefit by welcoming noble ideas from every one. The collective result of all noble ideas will do collective good. It is the pooling of the best minds and the best thoughts, which results in the best action. These ideas are easy to implement. There will not be negative thoughts to cause interruptions. Nor will there be any dissipation of energy. Openness of mind manifests in such cases for there is nothing to fear. Noble thoughts through noble ideas result in noble acts and by evolving a noble character bring noble results. For example, from a single thought of increasing food production the innovative method of increasing productivity originates. It raises food output substantially. It benefits several millions and the destiny of a nation changes from poverty to prosperity. On the contrary a single thought of destroying others with ideas and acts of deploying destructive weapons ultimately result in the loss of several lives. The examples of 9/11 calamity and world wars make this clear.

Knowledge is power. It can be right knowledge or destructive knowledge. Whether knowledge is right or destructive depends on the ideas fed into the brain for assimilation. We witness knowledge explosion and the growth of the knowledge industry. The question arises whether we should develop knowledge, which is beneficial to society or destructive. Everyone will say we should do the former. The inventions in medicines are the result of noble ideas and they benefit millions of people. An individual can devote his attention to screen ideas and entertain noble ones only. But as a nation responsibility for protecting the life and property of the citizens devolves on the government. So fully knowing that, an idea to invent a deadly destructive defensive weapon system may be necessary. Knowledge explosion has to be in the direction of what is good for the individual and for society.

The greater the content of noble ideas in a person, organization or government, the nobler will be the benefits to society. If a nation or individual devotes the entire energy for designing weapons of destruction with the strategy to accomplish it then only evil results will follow. Positive thinking benefits the individual and society.

Negative thinking destroys both. The more the number of people and countries has noble thoughts and ideas the world becomes a better place to live. If it is the other way the world will be a palace of pain despite all progress and comforts we have achieved. All individuals developing noble thoughts and ideas collectively can make a better world. That should be the global perspective. There will be peace and happiness and we will be able to eliminate poverty, ensure happiness and welfare for all.

Those who develop noble thoughts and acts will find joy in giving and sharing with others what they have. The rich and well off sections of society should come forward to give part of their earnings to the poorer sections of the people without government intervention. If this is done globally a serious dent on the problem of poverty can be made. The hand of the giver is always higher. We can give anything, which is useful, or others. It can be materials of all types or knowledge, which will make them better and useful citizens. Giving knowledge is an enriching experience. It is like lighting several lamps from a single lamp. The mother lamp does not lose its brightness or light when the others are lighted. Similarly when all give to one another there will be love, happiness and prosperity. Problems will be less and effort and energy will be available for achieving great things. We can thus alleviate poverty and eliminate suffering to a greater extent.

When rich nations are achieving higher levels of living, poor nations are unable to maintain even the existing levels. They find the gap between needs and resources widening. In this context the views expressed by the famous economist and Nobel Laurite, Jan Tinbergen is of great significance.

"Generally the rich of the earth should prepare themselves for a simpler life in the future. The leading philosophy of the present, which always asks for more material goods and does not attach much value at simplicity of life or modesty in claims, has to be replaced by alternative philosophies and surely much could be learned from Mahatma Gandhi's words and example. The real values of life do contain a sufficient quantity of food and shelter; but it is not necessary to have the luxuries now aimed at. Cultural values will have to be "upgraded" again. The tremendous waste of armament and outer space research should be curtailed."

It is useful to remember the maxim:

Sow a thought and reap an idea,
Sow an idea and reap an act,
Sow an act and reap a character
Sow a character and reap a destiny.

Let us imbibe the content of this maxim and strive hard to achieve progress based on positive thoughts.

9. Learn from Nature-

We talk a lot about our planet's environment and its sustainability disregarding innumerable problems we create for mankind. Pollution levels all over the world are increasing. The urgency of the need to protect the environment is realized. Trees form a major part of the environment rendering us great service and benefits. They give us shade. They block clouds at high altitudes, condense water vapors and cause rains. They teach us useful lessons. Take the example of the banyan tree.

The banyan tree grows tall and has a large spread and its branches cover an area of more than an acre in some cases. It lives up to 400 years. It provides an air conditioning effect under its umbrella of branches free of cost. It cools the temperature in the vicinity giving shade and shelter. Its longevity reminds us of the several generations of men and women who have passed under its shade, probably a record no other tree enjoys.

From the huge banyan tree fall several seeds. Each seed, almost invisible to the naked eye contains great potential for bringing out several trees of even larger size to provide service to humanity. A small kernel of this tree contains thousands of seeds and has potential to give us off springs to cover the entire planet over thousands of years.

The banyan tree and the human mind have similarities. The mind is a subtle faculty. It is a flow of thoughts rushing through. These thoughts through ideas have potential for actions. If we screen them and take at least a few for scrutiny, development and implementation we find the basis for creative work in several fields. The nobler the idea the greater is the benefit for humanity.

The seeds of the banyan tree germinate under favorable environment and conditions. Similarly the human mind can germinate ideas under favorable conditions. We have to nurture the sapling with water, manure and care. Similarly we have to cultivate the mind for making it creative and productive. We as individuals or collectively as society have to provide the conditions for its development. If we do that just like the banyan tree we will be inclined to do only good to humanity. No wonder this tree is worshipped in countries like India.

It is educative to impress on our children this great contribution of the banyan tree and the lessons we can learn from it urging them to make their contribution to the welfare of society. They can make a beginning by planting a banyan sapling. They will learn to love and serve others like the banyan tree which offers shade and comfort to all without discrimination.

Modern management can learn a least one good lesson from the banyan tree. The example of the banyan tree helps us to develop a conceptual approach to problems. It teaches us to treat all employees with the same consideration and love. Business can grow with social responsibility which the banyan tree silently does.

In our daily life we don't have to go to any educational institutions to learn the fundamentals of human conduct and approach to life. If we observe nature manifesting through several forms of existence and living beings, we have ample material to learn and benefit. All that is needed is a keen sense of observation and discriminating intellect to grasp and assimilate. Here are a few examples.

The sun is the visible god to everyone. It is the source of all energy essential for life on this planet. It gives us heat and light. Just imagine our existence without the sun. It does not discriminate in distributing its benefits. It gives light to all living beings. It brings about climate changes and we have rains and sunshine. Crops grow and we get our food. All these are done without expecting anything in return. Do we show our gratitude to the sun? At least can we not pray to the sun god for all kindness shown, with reverence?

Next let us take the case of air. It purifies everything. It radiates the scent of flowers to us and gives a pleasant feeling without destroying them. At the same time it is no way affected by the scent. It is unaffected by the perfume or foul odor. It contains oxygen which is essential for our existence. Can we exist without oxygen even for two minutes? How long can you hold your breath?

You know how much we have to pay for a cylinder of oxygen to last ten minutes. At that rate how much should we pay if someone were to charge for the air we breathe in a life time? It is mind boggling. Instead what we do is to pollute the air by releasing all obnoxious gases, fumes and dust, making life difficult, miserable and unhealthy. We are inviting diseases because of our indifference to keep the air free from pollution.

Now we come to fire. It is available everywhere. it facilitates our cooking. It gives us warmth when we face adverse climate. It is the visible source of energy. It helps us to manufacture and process thousands of goods and services for our living. But if carelessly handled, it causes death and destruction. We have to respect it. Forest fires and inferno cause widespread havoc. This is because of our neglect and disrespect to fire.

Now let us consider space. Can we move an inch forward or backward without space? It is not polluted in any way. Everything exists in space. Without space we cannot think of existence of anything. But do we recognize this great boon in our daily life. Just imagine if we have to pay a fee every time for covering a few feet of distance. How much we will have to pay and can we afford it?

Water is another gift without which we cannot live. It purifies and cleans everything. It is the medium for our cleanliness and processing of food. It facilitates navigation. Without it we cannot survive.

Then we consider the earth. How patient the earth is. We overburden it by building several billion tons of structures on it. We dig the earth several times in several places. We dump all filth in it. But it never complains. Is there anything greater than Mother Earth to teach us patience? Do we ever recognize this and pay our homage to it.

The cow is another example of an animal of service to man. It gives us milk and manure. Its hides, skin and bones are useful for making several articles. To such an animal what do we give? We give fodder which is the unwanted remnant of the crops we grow. By accepting this cow continues to serve man. Is it not a great act of generosity on the part of cow which gives the most nutritious item without expecting anything in return? Is it not an example of patience and great service?

These are a few examples of how man can learn from nature. Even objects and animals we consider to be insignificant do us great service and teach us valuable lessons to improve our approach to life and widen the horizon of our thinking and knowledge. Above all they teach us humility. Why not we live in harmony with them?

10. Facing Death:

It was Lord Francis Bacon who said," Men fear death just as children fear to walk in darkness." We all know that if there is one thing with 100% certainty in this world it is death, which does not make any exception. People having realized the inevitability of this event become panicky while entertaining thoughts of death. This event of change occurs in all living organisms after undergoing various stages as birth, growth, decay, and disease. Death caps all these and dispenses with the body once for all. The organs gradually weaken and after becoming non responsive to even the most modern medicines, surrender totally to the phenomenon of death. The same body, which once was nurtured, cared and protected, now becomes redundant and looks horrible demanding immediate removal and disintegration.

This happens when the body faces internal decay due to disease inherent in the decomposition of properties encased in it. Decay also occurs due to severe damage caused by impact of external forces like accidents, natural calamities and the like. There is no age limit for this event to occur. What we can say is in the case of normal individuals with healthy life styles the aging process can be postponed and the organs maintained in fairly healthy and functioning condition for a longer duration. This does not in any way guarantee endless protection or prolonging existence. The biological system within the body no longer is fit to resist the invading viruses, bacteria and threats so that the body gives away and falls dead motionless. This becomes inevitable. No power on earth can make it move further even for a minute in the natural way. Ultimately the body is consigned to flames or buried deep under the earth to decompose and merge with the basic elements from which the Universe has originated.

Death occurs when external and internal forces threaten the body in several ways bringing about its annihilation. One who has wasted deliberately or otherwise all his mental intellectual and physical strength invites death at an early stage compared to one who is very careful.

The body dies and not the spirit. To analyze and understand death it is relevant and useful to differentiate between the body and the invisible spirit, which according to Hinduism, never is born or never dies, which has no beginning or end. It is a spark of the great Divinity we all know as the Supreme Consciousness. The body, which becomes useless, due to decay and disease, is to be cast away like a torn shirt. It is a wonderful philosophy.

When the inevitable moment draws to a close, those who have semblance of memory will laugh at the futility of resisting death and in trying out alternatives to prolong ones existence. It is not worth the effort for the event overtakes all such attempts. So to face it boldly one has to be prepared. There should be full conviction that death is inevitable. No one could escape from its jaws. The earlier a person develops an attitude that he or she is not the body which alone is perishable and he or she is the spirit which pervades all living beings in the universe, the better. When this faith is deep rooted in one's thinking the person enters a stage of deathlessness. He always thinks of the spirit and is ready to cast away the body, which falls off like a ripened fruit effortlessly.

11. Love all

Let each one of us who are blessed and well off, make a humble beginning by helping at least one individual around us who is in dire need and for whom two meals a day is a luxury. If we succeed the world will be a better place to live for all. There will be universal peace and happiness. Is it not worth striving and attaining? We can definitely attain this state of happiness, with perseverance.

When are we going to realize that the most valuable and precious but essential things of life are free which. Nature has provided us in abundance. Space, air, water, heat are examples. We take them for granted but do not desist from our attempts to pollute or misuse them. A contented society with collective happiness is a goal worth attempting and achieving.

Life is full of joy and there is no reason to complain about anything. God has given us all that we need. Happiness cannot be purchased. It has to be lived and experienced within. It requires a philosophy and understanding one's limitations and the meaning of death, which every human being will pass through. The attitude rooted in spirituality considerably helps to face that eventuality also.

Detailed analysis of their problem and recasting of priorities can go a long way to solve the problems. If they are still dissatisfied, then the problem is within them and only a change in attitude can find a solution. Otherwise they create problems for which they alone are responsible.

It is like the case of a person who kills his parents and pleads for help saying he is an orphan. Such individuals are plagued by consumerism and are grossly materialistic. They have not taken refuge in spirituality which can make a sea change in their mental condition and ensure happiness. For those who don't try this simple and inexpensive method of being happy and thus free from complaints we can only sympathize with them .They forget to live though exist.

Can we not learn to be wise and give up pursuit of foolishness to avoid global calamity? Let us make a beginning to change our lifestyle by implanting that which will enrich, nourish our health and happiness.

: